The Cornea in Measles

Monographs in Ophthalmology 3

Dr W. JUNK PUBLISHERS THE HAGUE – BOSTON – LONDON

N. W. H. M. DEKKERS

The Cornea in Measles

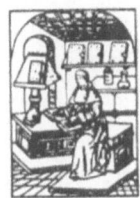

DR W. JUNK PUBLISHERS THE HAGUE – BOSTON – LONDON

Distributors:

for the United States and Canada
Kluwer Boston Inc.
190 Old Derby Street
Hingham, MA 02043
USA

for all other countries
Kluwer Academic Publishing Group
Distribution Center
P.O. Box 322
3300 AH Dordrecht
The Netherlands

ISBN-13: 978-94-009-8679-4   e-ISBN-13: 978-94-009-8677-0
DOI: 10.1007/978-94-009-8677-0

Preface

The need to study the corneal complications of measles was not very obvious. Everyone knew of the (kerato) conjunctivitis of measles and considered it to be an innocuous feature of the disease. Every medical worker in developing countries knew that measles in under- or malnourished children runs a very serious course leading to, e.g., corneal complications. The latter are seen frequently that medical workers in developing countries are in the habit of speaking of post-measles blindness. The aspect of the cornea in post-measles blindness is reminiscent of the keratomalacia in vitamine A deficiency and kwashiorkor. It was suggested that in measles the last reserves of vitamine A are exhausted, thereby precipitating the keratomalacia. The virological origin of measles keratitis has been more or less neglected in literature up till now.

This study provides clinical and laboratory data concerning the kerato-conjunctivitis of measles, gathered from a number of hospitalized children in a rural area of Kenya. The merits of this monograph is that it gives a careful description of the clinical course of measles keratoconjunctivitis and that it emphasizes the role of the virus-infection in addition to protein deficiency and vitamine A-deficiency in the etiology of post-measles blindness. The possible roles of exposure in semi-comatose patients and of the application of traditional autochthone medicine are mentioned. Measles is no longer seen in developed countries but will still be encountered in the developing countries. The measles-vaccination program is hampered by some problems in the preservation of the vaccin.

This monograph is the result of an unbiased outlook on the problem of corneal complications in measles and the reader who is not ignorant of conditions in rural hospitals in Africa cannot but admire the energy and the organizational talent that were devoted to the accomplishment of this project, in which the cooperation of laboratories in Nairobi, Rotterdam and Amsterdam was indispensable.

Contents

1 — Introduction

1.1. Blinding eye complications after measles: "Post-Measles-Blindness"

In several developing countries blindness after measles is a considerable public health problem. Many patients, who have lost useful vision through leucomata, adhaerent leucomata or phthisis bulbi, relate this with an episode of measles when they were young. For example, in a survey in Western Kenya of two Schools for the Blind, I found a prevalence of 30% for corneal blindness, and the majority of these children blamed the measles. (unpublished data; cfr Sauter 1976).

It seemed unjustified to me, to connect the corneal blindness after measles with a single, specific pathogenetic mechanism, e.g. Vitamin A dependant keratomalacia. For this reason the more comprehensive term "Post-Measles-Blindness" (PMB) is preferred. This indicates the relation in time between measles and the subsequent blindness, and permits study of the problem without prejudice.

In addition to a high prevalence in blindness statistics (§ 2.7) a high incidence of PMB is currently reported in studies of measles from developing countries. Kimati and Lyaruu (1976) reported 5 cases with corneal involvement leading to blindness out of 624 patients with measles, admitted to the Mwanza Regional Hospital, Tanzania. Ophthalmological details are not available. 44 Out of 2,376 (1.9%) measles patients, reported by Morley, Martin and Allen (1967) in East-Africa, developed permanent ocular damage. In this study ocular damage was associated with a high mortality (cfr Animashaun 1977).

Similar reports are published from West-Africa: 31 out of 2,164 patients (1.4%) with destruction of one or both eyes (Morley 1969) and 27 cases of corneal blindness out of 2,772 measles-patients (1.0%) in Lagos, Nigeria (Animashaun 1977).

These statistics make it likely, that in at least some African countries in development, somewhere around 1% of all children with measles will sustain permanent, severe ocular damage of corneal origin.

Ocular complications in measles are not necessarily localized in the cornea. Retrobulbar neuritis (Srivastava and Nema 1963) and retinitis (Bücklers 1969; Haydn 1970; Regensburg and Henkes 1976) are described, but in developing countries these are rare compared to the corneal complications. In this study only the corneal involvement with measles will be taken into account.

1.2. Pathogenesis of Post-Measles-Blindness

In the literature on PMB 3 possible pathogenetic pathways can be identified: infection, malnutrition and treatment. In chapter 2 a detailed review of the literature will be given. In this section only the outlines will be given, as far as they are needed to define the purpose of this study.

a. Infection

Occasionally a coarse punctate keratitis is mentioned as a sign of measles (Trantas 1903; Thygeson 1959); severe corneal damage, however, is seldom attributed to the measles virus itself: Frederique, Howard and Boniuk (1969) are the exception.

A herpetic keratitis was seen early in the measles infection (Sauter 1976) and Whittle et al. (1979) were able to culture herpes simplex virus from corneal ulcers after measles.

An unspecified bacterial superinfection is, however, considered as a more important possibility by many authors (Gaud 1958; Armengaud et al. 1961; Quéré 1964; Benezra and Chirambo 1977).

No report on fungal infections of the cornea in connection with PMB was found.

b. Malnutrition

Protein Energy Malnutrition (PEM) and morbidity from measles go hand in hand: measles runs a more severe course in malnourished children (Scheifele and Forbes 1973) and overt kwashiorkor is a frequent complication of measles (Kimati and Lyaruu 1976; Alleyne et al. 1977). The deep disturbance of the protein metabolism in PEM might in itself be a reason for the necrosis of the cornea (Moore 1957; McLaren 1963; Kuming and Politzer 1967).

Most attention however has been given to the disturbance of Vitamin A metabolism in measles. The intake of Vitamin A and its precursors is reduced with grossly reduced food intake. The absorption is diminished because of diarrhoea. The serum levels of retinol and Retinol Binding Protein (RBP) are lowered because of infection and fever (Moore 1957; Morley, Woodland and Martin 1963; Arroyave and Calcaño 1979; Axton 1979). This reduced availability of Vitamin A, alone, or in combination with PEM, is held responsible for a Vitamin A dependant keratomalacia in the wake of measles (Oomen, McLaren and Escapini 1964). In this view, measles is only the trigger to produce a manifest keratomalacia in a previously only marginally deficient child.

c. Treatment

In the ophthalmological literature originating in Africa much attention is given to the possible role of traditional medicines. Vivid descriptions of their use can be found (Phillips 1961).

They are widely in use in Africa (Ayanru 1974; Kokwaro 1976; Chirambo and Benezra 1976; Maina-Ahlberg 1979). Some of the vegetable materials in use as ocular medicines can cause corneal damage. (Crowder and Sexton 1964; Cordero-Moreno 1973). The significance attached to their use is contro-versial and varies from "nonsense" (McManus 1968) to "the most important" cause of Post-Measles-Blindness (Phillips 1961).

In tropical countries childhood morbidity and mortality are considerable. Measles is not the only disease severely afflicting the under-fives in under-priviliged conditions. It shares its bad reputation with malaria, pneumonia, gastro-enteritis, whooping cough and tuberculosis. But still, of these diseases measles especially is extremely frequently mentioned as a factor connected with corneal blindness, originating in childhood.

This clinical observation suggests that the cornea is intrisically involved with measles: measles might directly affect the cornea.

The previously mentioned pathogenetic pathways take this connection insufficiently into account and the question remains: why does Post-Measles-Blindness occur? To answer this question it is first of all necessary to know what happens to the cornea in the acute stage of measles.

1.3. Lack of knowledge about the cornea in early measles

The question about corneal involvement in measles may look selfevident, but remarkably little attention has been paid to this subject: the literature is very scanty and gives only few ophthalmological details.

In 1903 Trantas (Constantinople) describes for the first time a punctate keratitis as a sign of measles. The existence of this keratitis is — among others — confirmed by Thygeson (1959), but very few detailed descriptions are to be found.

Even less attention has been given to the early corneal complications of measles.

Also in the limited amount of literature on the corneal signs of the acute stage of measles no connection is made with possibly blinding complications. The statement of Quéré (1964) "Ophthalmology has neglected measles" still holds true.

1.4 Purpose and content of the present study

The involvement of the cornea in the acute stage of measles is the subject of the present study. The best study on the measles-keratitis now available is still the one by Trantas in 1903. It seems wo thwhile therefore to study this self-limiting keratitis with the investigative tools now available. The attention paid to this keratitis is above all warranted by the possible occurrence of blinding complications: the existence of Post-Measles-Blindness (1% in developing countries) is the incentive for this study.

It is hoped that by the study of the early corneal signs of measles, some data relevant for the pathogenesis of PMB can be obtained, which hopefully might have implications for the prevention of PMB.

In the background of every infection, the nutritional status of the child is the most important, not to say the decisive factor for the final outcome of the disease. It is even said that "a community is malnourished so long as children die of measles" (King et al. 1972). In the literature PMB is also invariably connected with Protein Energy Malnutrition (P.E.M.)(Rodger 1959; Oomen, McLaren and Escapini 1964). Complications are associated with PEM, but the possibility exists that also the severity of physical signs is influenced by the nutritional status (O'Donovan 1971; Dossetor, Whittle and Greenwood 1977). In this study much attention is therefore given to the possible association of corneal disease with the nutritional status.

In the literature on measles the terms signs, symptoms and complications are used indiscriminately to describe anything that is observed on the cornea. For the purpose of this study physical signs and symptoms are defined as any phenomenon related to the multiplication of the measles virus and the normal reaction of the healthy body against this viral invasion. Anything beyond this interaction constitutes a complication. According to these definitions the Koplik's spots and the rash are signs, buccal ulcers are complications.

In chapter 4 a detailed description of the conjunctival and corneal *signs* of measles will be given and in chapter 6 it will be demonstrated that these signs are independent of the nutritional status of the affected children.

It is, however, in no way the purpose of this study to deny the association of blinding *complications* after measles with the nutritional status (i.e. Protein Energy Malnutrition and/or Vitamin A Deficiency). Nor will it be possible to derive from this study any conclusion -- positive or negative -- about the prevalence of Vitamin A Deficiency in the population. The subject of this study is measles.

This study was mainly done in a 150 bed rural mission hospital in Western Kenya. Here in a two year period 248 children, acutely ill with measles were followed by daily slitlamp examination. They all had an anthropometric assessment of their nutritional status. Serum samples were analysed in Nairobi (400 km away); conjunctival specimens for immunofluorescence and electron-microscopy were sent to The Netherlands.

A rural mission hospital and a governmental Provincial Hospital are hardly equipped for research purposes. But, because of the motivation for this study (PMB in under-priviliged conditions) it had to be done somewhere in the bush. This gave much difficulty in getting things organised, and done. This work would never had been carried out if I hadn't had the enthusiastic support and cooperation of so many others. I owe them many thanks.

2 – Review of literature

2.1. The epidemiology of measles

In developing countries measles is a public health problem of considerable importance, because of its high prevalence in combination with a high mortality rate.

In Kenya measles is an endemic disease, with an epidemic outbreak every 2(−3) years (cfr Morley, Woodland and Martin (Nigeria) 1963; Voorhoeve et al. 1977) Nearly all children get measles, and, compared to Europe, at a relatively early age (8--36 months). This is probably caused by the over-crowding of the African households, resulting in a higher infection load at this early age (Leary and Obst 1966).

The mortality for measles is high. In hospital statistics the case fatality rate is 8.6% (Bwibo 1970) to 25% (Morley 1969) and is usually presented to be about 15- 20%. In field studies however the mortality rate is under-standably lower: 6.8% in Nigeria (Morley, Woodland and Martin 1963), 6.5% in a Kenyan study (Voorhoeve et al. 1977). The West African saying "count your children after the measles" needs no further explanation.

The mortality can vary considerably in different epidemics (Muller et al. 1977). The lower age of infection is accompanied by a higher mortality (Bwibo 1970; O'Donovan 1971; Cruickshank, Standard and Russell 1976) and is highest in the age-group of 1−2 years (Voorhoeve et al. 1977). According to many studies this higher mortality could be caused by the higher frequency of undernutrition in the lower age groups (Leary and Obst 1966; Morley, Martin and Allen 1967; O'Donovan 1971; Hendrickse 1975; Dossetor, Whittle and Greenwood 1977; Muller et al. 1977).

Also the morbidity from measles is considerable: the accompanying stomatitis, laryngotracheitis and gastroenteritis may be severe, whereas bronchopneumonia, otitis media, and Protein Energy Malnutrition are fre-quent complications (Leary and Obst 1966; Bwibo 1970; Kimati and Lyaruu 1976). It has been mentioned already in §1.1. that 1% of the measles children sustain permanent ocular damage.

Early this century the same situation existed in Western Europe. For example, in 1908 in Glasgow 5.8% of the under-fives infected with measles died (Morley, Woodland and Martin 1963). In Europe measles has now become a benign disease (in Great Britain the case fatality rate is 1:10,000 (Cruickshank, Standard and Russell, 1976) because of the socio-economic development, rather than the introduction of modern medicine. The differences in the epidemiology of measles, in Europe and developing countries, can be explained on non-geographical grounds. These differences are associated with socio-economic and cultural differences, not with dif-ferent climates or different strains of the measles-virus. There are therefore no reasons to consider "Tropical measles" a separate entity. The use of this

10

term is to be dropped (cfr Cruickshank, Standard and Russell 1976; Muller et al. 1977; Benezra and Chirambo 1978).

2.2. The extra- and intracellular morphology of the measles virus

The measles virus belongs -- together with the viruses of rinderpest and canine distemper -- to the group of pseudomyxoviruses. They share a common morphology and some cross-immune reactions (Wilterdink 1979).

The virion measures 120–300 nm. (1 nanometer = 10^{-9} m) on electron-microscopical examination, but only 100 nm. in filtration experiments. It is polymorph in shape and occasionally anomalous and long filamentous forms can be seen.

Pseudomyxoviruses have a lipoprotein envelope, on which numerous spikes, 10 nm. in length, are visible. The envelope itself has also a thickness of 10 nm. (fig. 2.2.a). A unit of nucleocapsid of measles virus consists of RNA combined with a protective protein. About 2000 of these units are wound into a single helix, where the RNA as the carrier of genetic material is surrounded and protected by the protein. The diameter of this helix is 18 nm., the pitch of the helix is 4.5 nm. (fig. 2.2.b).

The overall length in electronmicroscopical specimens, stained with negative contrast, is approximately 1000 nm. Inside the lipoprotein-envelope the nucleocapsid helix is haphazardly folded. (Hall and Martin 1975; Wilterdink 1979).

The measles virion makes contact with the receptor sites at the surface of

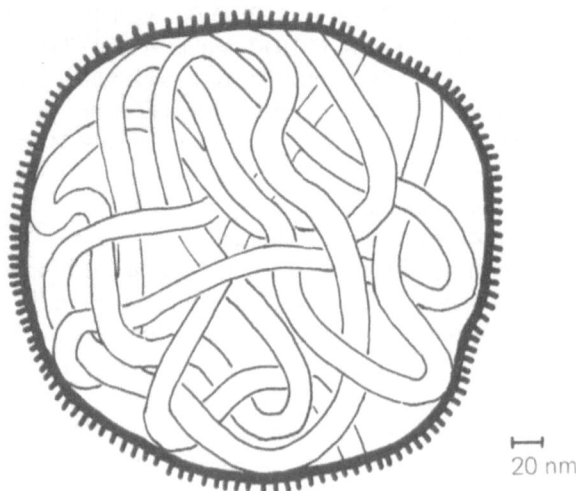

20 nm

Figure 2.2.a. The morphology of the complete virion, the appearance of the extra-cellular measles-virus

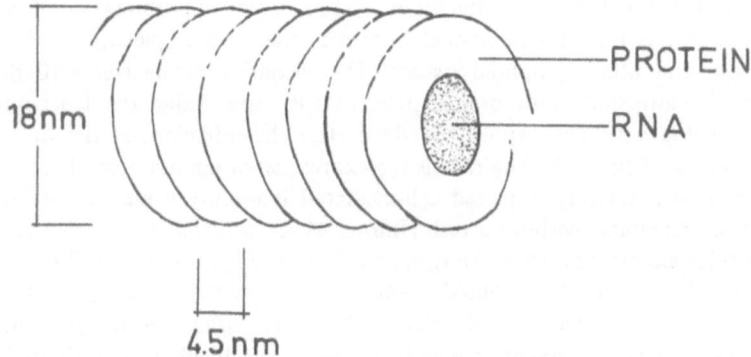

Figure 2.2.b. The ultrastructure of the RNA strands within the virion. Inside the infected cells these strands are present without the protective envelope (cfr fig 5.2.3.g.)

the host cell. The envelope merges with the cell membrane and the viral nucleocapsid is taken into the cytoplasm. With the use of the metabolism of the hostcell, RNA re-duplication commences with the formation of a viral messenger-RNA. Later on newly formed RNA is combined with the protecting proteins to form the helical nucleocapsid. These nucleocapsids are located in inclusion bodies, visible 16–20 hours after the infection in the cytoplasm, 96–120 hours after the infection inside the nucleus (Morgan and Rapp 1977).

The newly formed nucleocapsid induces a change in the cellular membrane, visible as a higher density on electronmicroscopic examination. In a "budding process" the altered cellular membrane, with newly induced haemadsorption properties, engulfs the nucleocapsid and subsequently forms the envelope. The now complete virions are set free into the intercellular fluids, and continue on their way to the next cells (Nakai and Imagawa 1969; Wilterdink 1979).

The virion is thus the extracellular, the nucleocapsid helix the intracellular morphological appearance of the measles virus.

2.3. The pathogenesis of the measles infection

The first contact with the highly infective virus is at the mucous membrane of the respiratory tract. Also the conjunctiva might act as a portal of entry for the measles infection (Papp 1954). If not inactivated by mucus or specific secretory IgA antibodies (Dawson 1976) the virus enters the ciliated columnar epithelium and a small focus is located in the oro-pharynx, where it is hardly ever detected. Where the conjunctiva is the portal of entry, a "conjunctivitis of infection" may be the clinical result. During the primary viraemia, 2–6 days after the infection, the virus is transported intracellularly inside the formed elements of the blood. Macrophages withdraw most of the virus and debris of infected cells from the blood, and an extensive proliferation of virus follows in the reticulo-endothelial system in the tonsils, spleen, liver, bone-marrow and other lymphoid tissues. The second viraemia starts 10 days after the infection, with proliferation of the virus inside the leucocytes. Neutralizing antibodies appear 14 days after the infection, at the time of appearance of the rash. The rash is the expression of immunological defense: in cases with severely impaired cell-mediated immunity a measles-infection may run its course without a rash (Burnet 1968; Scheifele and Forbes 1973; cfr Cruickshrank et al. 1974; Morgan and Rapp 1977; Wilterdink 1979).

The formation of lymphoid giant cells (Finkeldey-Warthin cells) is a characteristic cytopathogenetic effect of measles virus. The demonstration of their presence in tissues or secretions can be a valuable diagnostic sign of prodromal measles. They are however present in only half of all measles cases (Roberts and Bain 1958).

The virus is eliminated by humoral and cell-mediated immune responses: in most cases it will not be possible to culture the virus from the blood later than 36 hours after the outbreak of the rash.

The conjunctiva is involved in this pathogenetic process in two ways: as a possible portal of entry for the infection and the development of a characteristic conjunctivitis in the prodromal stage of measles. The potential importance of the conjunctiva as a portal of entry for measles has been demonstrated by Papp (1954, 1956, 1957), who found experimentally that, in the contact with measles patients, protection of the eyes with either goggles or anti-measles-convalescent serum dropped into the eyes, prevented the infection. When the primary focus of the measles infection is located in the conjunctiva, a "conjunctivitis of infection" may be the result (Goodall, in Grist 1950; Robbins 1962).

The superficial layer of the lamina propria of the conjunctiva is made up of lymphoid tissue. Also in this tissue, a multiplication of the measles virus takes place after the first viraemia, and a manifest conjunctivitis is the clinical result.

This is the conjunctivitis, characteristic for the prodromal stage of measles.

2.4. Ocular signs and complications in measles

2.4.1. The conjunctivitis of infection

When the conjunctiva is the portal of entry for the measles infection, a "conjunctivis of infection" may be the result. (Herrman 1914; Goodall cited in Grist 1950; Robbins 1962). The practical importance of this observation is limited and bears no relation with the subject of the present study.

2.4.2. The conjunctivitis in prodromal measles.

A catarrhal conjunctivitis of variable extent is a characteristic sign of measles (cfr Gemert, Valkenburg and Muller 1977) and has a high diagnostic value. In accordance with the pathogenesis of the measles-infection, this conjunctivitis has a subepithelial localization.

The conjunctival epithelium can be involved too. Occasionally lesions comparable to Koplik's spots can be observed. When localized at the caruncula or the semilunar fold they are of diagnostic value (Bonamour 1953; Gaud 1958; Nataf, Lépine and Bonamour 1960; Fedukowicz 1978). Very rarely vesicles with a contagious content are found in the conjunctival epithelium (Bonamour 1953b).

Azizi and Krakovsky (1965) observed in the majority of their measles cases — on slitlamp examination and using fluorescein 2% eyedrops — lesions of the conjunctival epithelium, continuous with similar lesions in the corneal epithelium. These epithelial lesions were localized in the palpebral slit. They were strictly epithelial, without subepithelial infiltration or other signs of inflammation. These authors state explicitly that this keratoconjunctivitis is a sign, not of a complication, of measles.

These same lesions were observed by Sauter (1976), their presence could be demonstrated with the use of the vital stains Rose Bengal and Lissamine Green. Because of these staining properties Sauter (1976) considered these epithelial lesions as signs of Vitamin A deficiency.

For the purpose of the present study it will be very important to know whether these lesions are of viral origin or induced by Vitamin A deficiency. Much attention will therefore be given to the immunofluorescence and electronmicroscopy of conjunctival biopsies (§ 5.1 and § 5.2.3) and the significance of the vital stains Lissamine Green and Rose Bengal (§ 3.4).

Complications of this conjunctivitis occur. An (unspecified) bacterial superinfection is possible; a combination with a diphtheric conjunctivitis is a rarity (Gaud 1958; Nataf, Lépine and Bonamour 1960).

Occasionally a phlyctenular keratoconjunctivitis is seen (Gaud 1958).

2.4.3. The epithelial keratitis in measles

In 1903, Trantas (Constantinople) described for the first time a coarse punctate, strictly epithelial keratitis as a sign of measles. This keratitis occurs at the time of the rash, is usually bilateral, gives remarkably little subjective symptoms and heals without sequelae.

The existence of this keratitis is mentioned by some other authors (Cosmettatos 1908; Armengaud et al. 1961; Quéré 1964; Franken 1974; Sauter 1976), but only a few give some more details (Florman and Agatston 1962; Azizi and Krakovsky 1965). This keratitis is supposed to be caused by the measles virus (Trantas 1903; Jones 1960; Thygeson 1961; Casanovas 1976; Morgan and Rapp 1977).

There is considerable discongruence as regards the incidence of this keratitis:

— 4% : Armengaud et al. (1961) Senegal

- 10% : Quéré (1964) Senegal
- 30% : Sauter (1976) Kenya
- 71% : Lagraulet and Bard (1967) Upper Volta
- 76% : Trantas (1903) Turkey.

Thygeson (1961, USA) even states that this keratitis can be observed in every measles patient, provided he is seen early enough in the disease. These differences in incidence can at least be partially explained by the differences in examination technique: the incidence is necessarily higher in longitudinal studies (Trantas, Thygeson) than when it concerns snapshot visits (Sauter).

Not all authors agree upon the duration of the keratitis, most agree that it vanishes within days, without sequelae. Azizi and Krakovsky (1965) mention a duration of some weeks, whereas in the description of Florman and Agatston (1962) it may take the cornea some months to clear up.

It was already mentioned (§ 2.4.2) that Azizi and Krakovsky (1965) observed a continuity between the lesions in the corneal and conjunctival epithelium.

Central exfoliations of the corneal epithelium of larger size than the lesions of the coarse punctate keratitis of Trantas, were described by Förster and Berger (1892, cited in Trantas, 1903). This paper was not available in its original form. No other description of these central exfoliations could be traced.

2.4.4. Corneal ulcers, a complication of measles

The development of stromal ulcers is a complication of measles. These corneal ulcers have no particular morphological characteristics and are therefore indistinguishable from most other causes of corneal ulceration.

Usually a rim of normal corneal tissue is still present at the limbus. Perforation is common, the end result of these ulcers is a more or less dense leucoma, adhaerent leucoma or phthisis bulbi.

The leucomata are preferentially localized at the lower half of the cornea. Two explanations for this occurrence at the 6 o'clock position are given. Phillips (1961) (Zambia) mentions that when traditional medicines that hurt are applied to the eye, the eye is turned away (upward) as forcibly as possible and only the lower part of the cornea is exposed to the possibly noxious substances.

Sandford-Smith and Whittle (1979) (Nigeria) state that exposure and drying of the exposed cornea is an important pathogenetic factor in the cause of corneal ulceration after measles.

In this respect it may be of importance that Oomen (1961) distinguishes two different clinical forms of xerophthalmia: an acute total liquefaction of the cornea with extrusion of the contents of the eye and subsequent phthisis bulbi, and a more localized quiet perforation in the lower (or nasal) half of the cornea, resulting in a descemotocele and subsequently an adhaerent leucoma with the retention of at least some useful vision. This last form suggests the presence of a localizing factor.

However, much controversy exists as far as the pathogenetic interpretation of the ulceration is concerned. As mentioned earlier (§1.2) 3 main pathogenetic mechanisms can be identified: infection, malnutrition and treatment.

a. Infection

During a measles epidemic in Haiti, Frederique, Howard and Boniuk (1969) observed 25 children with corneal ulcers. In 14 patients the ulcers perforated, in 7 of them bilaterally. No signs of previous Vitamin A deficiency were present: no nightblindness, no xerosis, no Bitot's spots. Moreover, they mention "– the absence of any prior epidemic of nutritional keratomalacia with corneal perforation". Three eyes were examined histologically. The most prominent feature was the presence of multinucleate and syncytial cells in the epithelium, like those commonly seen in measles (cfr Scheifele and Forbes 1973). No specific changes in the corneal stroma were described. They concluded that the measles virus is to be held responsible for the corneal ulcers. Probably it is no coincidence that all 25 children were described as "markedly malnourished".

Bacterial superinfection is another possible cause of corneal ulceration. Armengaud et al. (1961) observed 14 corneal ulcera in 416 consecutive cases of measles. These ulcers developed from the fifth day onwards after the rash in an area of punctate keratitis. The authors consider secondary bacterial infection responsible for the ulcers (Thygeson 1957; Rodger 1959; Quéré et al. 1967; cfr Lagraulet and Bard 1967). No complications were seen, however, when topical antibiotics were administered routinely (Quéré 1964; Lagraulet and Bard 1967; Quéré et al. 1967; Muller et al. 1977).

A bacterial infection of the xerotic cornea (i.e. in cases of corneal xerophthalmia) might be another potential cause of severe corneal damage (Kuming and Politzer 1967; Sullivan, McCulley and Dohlman 1973).

Sandford-Smith and Whittle (1979) demonstrated the possibility of a viral superinfection (with the herpes simplex virus) in cases of corneal ulceration after measles.

The possibility exists that fungal infections are initiated by the instillation of traditional African medicines (Phillips 1961).

b. Malnutrition

If malnutrition is considered as the main cause of corneal ulceration after measles, a distinction is to be made between Vitamin A Deficiency (= xerophthalmia) and Protein Energy Malnutrition (PEM).

Xerophthalmia after measles is considered to be a frequent event (Oomen, McLaren and Escapini 1964; ten Doesschate 1968; Oomen J.M.V. 1971; Franken 1974; Sauter 1976). Van Manen (1938) noticed in Indonesia that an epidemic of measles is followed in its wake by an epidemic of xerophthalmia.

Xerophthalmia after measles occurs in the majority of cases in children without any previous clinical sign of Vitamin A deficiency (Oomen 1961). The diminished intake of Vitamin A and its precursors and the decreased bio-availability of retinol are the causes of this xerophthalmia occurring "out of the blue". Also a lack of the B-vitamins can be a cause of corneal disease. The "nutritional corneal dystrophy" in P.O.W.'s (Spyratos 1949; Petzetakis 1950; Alleyne et al. 1977) and the "malnutritional kerato-conjunctivitis" (Blumenthal 1950, 1960) are only mentioned here because of their connection with malnutrition. They have probably no relation to measles.

On the other hand, it is to be remembered that in nearly all cases with corneal complications encountered in the literature, the patients are invariably described as (markedly) malnourished. This has even led to the suggestion that keratomalacia might be a matter of PEM and not primarily of Vitamin A deficiency. (Yap-Kie-Tiong 1956; Arroyave et al. 1961; Reddy and Srikantia 1966; Venkataswamy 1967; Kuming and Politzer 1967; MacManus 1968; Emiru 1971; Baisya et al. 1971).

The observation that routine mass distribution of Vitamin A capsules (like in San Salvador and Indonesia) does prevent the minor forms of xero-phthalmia (nightblindness, xerosis and Bitot's spots) but not the kerato-malacia (Sommer, Faich and Quesada 1975; Pirie 1976), is an argument in the same direction.

c. Treatment

It has been mentioned in § 2.4.4.a that no corneal complications were observed when topical antibiotics were routinely applied to the eyes in cases of measles.

In contrast to the supposedly beneficial effect of these preparations, the use of topical traditional medicines could quite well be an important cause of blindness after measles. "During the prodromal stage of measles – irritant peppers and toxic substances are instilled in the eye as part of "traditional treatment". Corneal burns, ulceration, perforations and secondary infection lead to blindness." (Ayanru 1974.)

"Used in eyes, rendered more susceptible by existing pathology, the mechanical abrasive action of the powdered medication, the toxicity, acidity or alkalinity of the liquid preparations and the introduction of pathogens and fungi by the grossly unhygienic methods of preparation, must destroy countless corneae and eyes every year." (Phillips 1961.) (cfr McGlashan 1969; Jamieson 1970; Osuntokun 1975; Benezra and Chirambo 1977).

Strictly speaking, no proof is available about their harmful effects to the cornea, but "circumstantial evidence" (Agatha Christie) about their possible deleterious side-effects will be presented in a separate paragraph.

2.5. Depression of serumproteins, cell-mediated immunity and serum retinol in malnutrition

Serumproteins in malnutrition

Kwashiorkor and marasmus are the two extremes of the clinical spectrum of Protein Energy Malnutrition (PEM). Traditionally marasmus is supposed to be caused by the lack of food, providing the necessary energy, whereas kwashiorkor is attributed to a lack of protein. To explain the pathogenesis of kwashiorkor and clinical and epidemiological differences between kwashiorkor and marasmus, the concept of "disadaptation" was introduced (Waterlow and Payne 1975; Alleyne et al. 1977). In this view the marasmic child is chronically malnourished and uses its limited external energy sources in combination with katabolic mechanisms to maintain its biochemical equilibrium.

This adaptation mechanism fails in kwashiorkor (McLaren 1974; Waterlow and Payne 1975; Baily 1975; Eddy 1977). The balance between requirement and input is acutely disturbed (weaning, infection) and the child doesn't get the time to develop protective adaptive mechanisms, with all the clinical consequences of this failure. This concept explains why in marasmus the biochemical changes are minimal, whereas in kwashiorkor a profound biochemical disturbance exists (Whitehead, Coward and Lunn 1973).

One of the effects of the metabolic disturbance in kwashiorkor is the decrease in proteinsynthesis. The first proteins to be affected are some transport proteins with a rapid turnover, of which Retinol Binding Protein (RBP) is an example. The RBP level in the serum is therefore regarded as a fast reacting indicator of the impairement or improvement of the nutritional status (Ingenbleek et al. 1972, 1975a–b; Shetty et al. 1979).

The synthesis of serum albumin is also impaired, but at a much slower rate. The serum albumin is considered as a good, but slow, reacting indicator for the nutritional status. When the serum level of this protein drops below 3 gr%, biochemical deterioration sets in (Whitehead, Frood and Poskitt, 1971; Hay, Whitehead and Spicer, 1975). It is to be remembered however, that also measles itself is a cause for a lowering of the serum albumin level (Poskitt 1971).

The estimation of serum albumin and serum RBP therefore gives some information about the nutritional status of the child.

Immunological disturbance in malnutrition.

In general, malnutrition raises the susceptibility for infections (Emiru 1971), this holds especially true for bacterial infections (Scrimshaw, Taylor and Gordon 1959).

In malnutrition the infection, once established, also runs a more severe course. Mortality and morbidity increase considerably with increasing malnutrition (Geddes and Gregory 1974; Orren et al. 1979). This is caused by a depression of the cell mediated immunity in kwashiorkor and marasmus (Sellmeyer et al. 1972). This depression of cell mediated immunity might be more severe in kwashiorkor.

The same applies to measles in combination with malnutrition. In malnourished children a prolonged excretion of Finkeldey-Warthin cells in nasal secretions was found: 12 days compared to 3 days in "normal" measles (Scheifele and Forbes 1972).

The delay in, or qualitative impairment of, the cell-mediated-immunity could easily be the cause of a bigger virusload and therefore of viral complications (Enders et al. 1959; Scheifele and Forbes 1972; Whittle et al. 1979).

In cases of very severe depression of cell mediated immunity (caused by malnutrition or immunosuppression by other mechanisms) measles can run its course even without the development of a rash (Burnet 1968; cfr Kimura, Tosaka and Nakao 1975). A malnourished child can therefore have a measles infection which stays undiagnosed, because of the lack of a rash.

Malnutrition not only deeply influences the course of the measles infection, but is in itself also a common complication of measles. Measles is an important reason for the "disadaptation" and can provoke an overt malnutrition in previously borderline malnourished children (Kimati and Lyaruu 1976; Alleyne et al. 1977). So it was found in Uganda, that 26% of the admissions for kwashiorkor had an infection with measles less than six weeks before the admission (Hay, Whitehead and Spicer 1975).

Serum retinol

Traditional treatment of measles (and the general illness of the child) includes a reduction in the intake of all food, including Vitamin A and its precursors. Moreover, the diarrhoea of measles interferes with the absorption. Vitamin A is, however, stored in large quantities in the liver and a diminished intake is probably not the cause of an acute deficiency (Moore 1957; Morley, Woodland and Martin 1963).

In all measles cases the serum retinol level is lowered, but this is possibly an aspecific effect of the fever because of increased metabolism (Moore 1957).

In cases of Protein-Energy-Malnutrition (PEM), the Retinol-Binding-Protein (RBP) is also lowered due to a reduction in the synthesis of apo-RBP, the protein part of the molecule. Since retinol is not present in its free form in the serum, a low serum retinol can therefore be caused by either a lack of retinol or a failing protein synthesis or both (Muto et al. 1972; Arroyave et al. 1961).

This means that a low serum retinol is therefore not automatically an indicator for Vitamin A Deficiency, in the same sense that a reduced RBP is not automatically a proof for the presence of PEM. Much caution is therefore needed in the interpretation of these biochemical estimations.

2.6. Traditional ocular medicines

The use of traditional medicines is widely spread all over Africa (Rodger 1959; Phillips 1961; Imperato and Traoré 1969; Kokwaro 1976; Chirambo and Benezra 1976). They are used in practically any condition, and are also frequently combined with western medicine (Maina-Ahlberg 1979).

In the literature several substances, instilled into the eyes, could be traced. They were in use as a treatment for "sore eyes" in general, or measles eyes more specifically.

— Powders:	powdered cowrie shell (McLaren 1960a)
	powdered sugar candy (Holmes 1959; Chirambo and Benezra 1976)
	soot (Phillips 1961)
— Minerals:	copper stone (Phillips 1961)
	copper sulphate (Holmes 1959)
— Foodstuffs:	honey (Imperato and Traoré 1969)
	breastmilk (Ayanru 1978)
	orange juice (Imperato and Traoré 1969)
	egg yolk (Maina-Ahlberg 1979)
— Plants:	a great many varieties (Kokwaro 1976)
— Miscellaneous:	cow's urine (Animashaun 1977)
	aspirin tablets (Renkema, personal communcation)

It will be obvious that powders may damage the cornea for mechanical reasons, and on a damaged cornea infections easily supervene.

Much damage will be caused by the physical and chemical properties of the preparation used: alkalinity or acidity, temperature, osmolarity. Moreover, the medicines can be toxic: copper may etch the cornea, resulting in abrasions and leucomata (Duke Elder and MacFaul 1972) and many "fresh" cases of traditional treatment look like acid or alkali burns (Chirambo and Benezra 1976). In many cases this may result in extensive scarring and symblepharon, whereas in other cases the cornea melts away totally with prolapse of the uvea (Chrambo and Benezra 1976). Also the impossibility of dosing the working principle of these preparations (Okoth, personal communication) is an important factor in the pathogenesis of the deleterious side effects of traditional medicines.

Most traditional medicines are of vegetable origin. Powders, decoctions, extracts and ashes derived from roots, tubers, stems, leaves, twigs and flowers are in use. Kokwaro (1976) mentions 75 plants used as eye medicines in East Africa. Of these, 18 are used in cases of conjunctivitis; measles is not mentioned specifically. Most probably many more are to be found (cfr Kerharo and Bouquet 1948; Rodger 1959).

For the explanation of possible negative effects of these medicines the emphasis is on the toxic substances found in these plants, e.g.: oxalates, saponines, steroid-like substances and cyanogenic glucosides.

The crushed leaves of *Oxalis corniculata L.* are, under the local names of Awayo (Luo) and Nandwa (Abaluyha), used to cure infected eyelids (Kokwaro 1976). *Oxalis spp.* however are known to contain large quantities of oxalates (Lewis and Elvin-Lewis 1977) what can be the cause of corneal ulcers (Duke-Elder and MacFaul 1972).

Many vegetable extracts contain saponins,* which may have a "deleterious action on the cornea, causing –, in concentrated solutions, chemosis, ulcerative keratitis and opacification" (Duke-Elder and MacFaul 1972). These saponins are present, among others, in Euphorbiaceae. An accidental contact with the sap of *Euphorbia tirucalli L.* (pencil tree) or *E. lactea* (candelabra cactus) can cause a considerable kerato-conjunctivitis.

In experiments, especially dogs are susceptible to this toxic effect (Crowder and Sexton 1964; Cordero-Moreno 1973). In this context it is however remarkable that the juice from the leaves and stem of *E. hirta L.* is used as a traditional eye medicine (Kokwaro 1976).

Moreover, some saponins have steroid properties or are steroid precursors. They are present – among others – in *Dioscorea spp, Polygala spp* and *Smilax spp* (Lewis and Elvin-Lewis 1977). Of these, the leaves of *Dioscorea astericus Burkill, Polygala persicariifolia DC, P. stenopetala Klotzsch* and *Smilax kraussiani Meisn* are used as traditional eye medicines in East Africa (Kokwaro 1976). The presence of steroids explains their fame as anti-inflammatory agents, but is of course not always beneficial (cfr herpes simplex virus and measles, § 2.4.4.a).

Ilusa is the local Abaluyha name for *Ageratum conyzoides L.*, of which the juice from the leaves is used to treat sore eyes (Kokwaro 1976). It contains however a cyanogenic glucoside (Lewis and Elvin-Lewis 1977) and HCN is known to reduce the repair activity of damaged corneal epithelium (Buschke 1949). Also *Cassia mimosoides L.*, around Kakamega used as eyedrops, under the name of Masambu or Koinyama, contains cyanide.

It is also to be remembered that in cases of measles these preparations are used in severely ill children, with a reduced resistance, whose corneae are already damaged by a viral keratitis. A deleterious effect of these traditional medicines is therefore quite conceivable.

In general, the application of these preparations causes considerable pain. Logical thinking would therefore discard their use as harmful, but in primitive thinking the pain is considered as a proof of the strength of the medicine, and its use can therefore be continued, despite the apparent lack of therapeutic success (Phillips 1961). The use of these medicines might also explain the common localization of corneal ulcers at the 6 o'clock position on the cornea (Phillips 1961).

The action of the traditional medicines is of course not always only

---

*Saponins are neutral amorphous glucosides of vegetable origin, with considerable surface action. They act strongly on cellular membranes (Bakker 1940, Duke-Elder and MacFaul 1972).

detrimental. The anti-inflammatory effect of some saponin-containing species has been mentioned before. Another example is *Aloë barbadensis*, the extract of which contains chrysophanic acid, which is beneficial for the skin (Lewis and Elvin-Lewis 1977). It may also be the working principle in aloë extracts for the healing of corneal ulcers (Mortada et al. 1976). On the other hand, chrysophanol is supposed to cause a chemotic conjunctivitis, keratitis and ulcers (Duke-Elder and MacFaul 1972). This difference might also be a matter of dosage. Too little is known about the effect of traditional medicines, their chemistry, toxicology and pharmacology. More attention is to be given to their use, especially in otherwise unexplainable conditions.

2.7. Statistics on Post-Measles-Blindness

In *Europe* Post-Measles-Blindness (PMB) is quantitatively unimportant. At a low overall blindness rate of 0.055% in the Netherlands, only 1% is related to measles. Corneal and posterior segment diseases are evenly represented (Schappert-Kimmijser 1959). The same was found in England (Fraser and Friedmann 1967) and Sweden (Lindstedt 1969).

In most blindness statistics from developing countries morphological and etiological criteria are mixed up and one has to be extremely careful to try to avoid a bias in the interpretation of these single sided blindness statistics.

In *Asia* the accent is on Vitamin A deficiency. In Serawak (Indonesia) 15 out of 103 patients, blinded below the age of 21 years, lost useful vision through keratomalacia "triggered" by measles. The same was found in 30% of the blind patients in Vietnam and South Korea (Oomen, McLaren and Escapini 1964).

Ten Doesschate (1968) describes in great detail the causes of blindness around Surabaya (Indonesia), in 675 blind children 285 cases of kerato-malacia were found. Only in 5 children measles was considered to be the principal cause of blindness, but in a considerable percentage of the kerato-malacia cases measles was the predisposing factor.

Africa

Rodger (1959) reported on the causes of blindness in North Nigeria, North Ghana and The Cameroons. Of the 193 blind children below the age of 10 years, 43 were blinded by measles; 17 were blinded by Vitamin A deficiency.

140 blind children were examined at the University Eye Clinic, Ibadan, Nigeria; 20 of them were blinded by measles (Olurin 1970). In 41 of the 116 enucleated eyes of children below the age of 10 years the corneal necrosis was associated with measles (Olurin 1973).

Also in Malawi 12% of childhood blindness is attributed to measles. One third of the inmates of the "Schools for the Blind" lost eyesight below the age of 3 years due to measles (Chirambo and Benezra 1976; Benezra and Chirambo 1977).

The figures from Zambia are even higher: of 686 blind persons, 64% blame measles as the cause of their blindness (McGlashan 1969).

Phillips (1961), also reporting from Zambia, states that even as much as 80% of blindness is caused by measles. He adds, however: "It is my firm conviction, that... African traditional medicines are the overwhelming cause of these lesions."

On the contrary, Blumenthal (1954) considers measles in South Africa a neglectable cause of blindness. The major cause of blindness (214 out of 895) is — what he calls — "malnutritional keratitis". This "discrete colliquative necrosis" (McLaren 1960b) is supposed to be caused by lack of the B-Vitamins (Blumenthal 1950, 1960). From these statistics it is evident that PMB is a considerable problem, surely, in Africa.

Kenya

Some statistics on the causes of blindness in Kenya are available. Sauter (1976) surveyed the "Schools for the Blind" and found that 352 of the 749 inmates (47%) had lost their eyesight due to xerophthalmia in "approximately 60%" of the cases in connection with measles. This high prevalence of corneal blindness in "Schools for the Blind" is in concordance with my own findings. Roughly one third of the childhood blindness, as found in these schools, is of corneal origin, one third relates to cataracts (frequently combined with microphthalmus) and one third is attributable to other, mainly congenital or neurological, causes.

These figures, however, don't give an indication of the overall prevalence of Post Measles Blindness, for which population-based surveys are needed.

The first survey for the causes of blindness in Kenya was conducted by Calcott (1956). 1093 Blind persons were examined: 183 showed a panophthalmitis, 182 corneal ulcers or their sequelae were encountered. No etiological diagnosis is given.

A number of random-sample surveys were done in several ethnic groups in Kenya.

Sinabulya (1976) examined 895 persons who had lost a total of 138 eyes, only one eye was lost in connection with measles. This study was done in Machakos, where also the "Joint Project Machakos" of the Medical Research Centre is going on. In this last study, with its emphasis on Mother and Child Care, not a single eye was lost because of measles. In this respect it is to be noted that Machakos, as far as medical care is concerned, is to be considered as a modern area (Muller et al. 1977; cfr Morley, Woodland and Martin 1963). Of the other surveys the numbers are not yet available.

3 – Patients and methods

3.1. Places and time

The provincial hospital at Kakamega is the referral centre for the district hospitals in Western Province, Kenya (see map 3.1). Specialist medical care is available only at this central facility.

The Provincial Ophthalmologist however, has his location at the St. Elizabeth Hospital Mukumu, a 150 bed Mission Hospital, 12 km South of

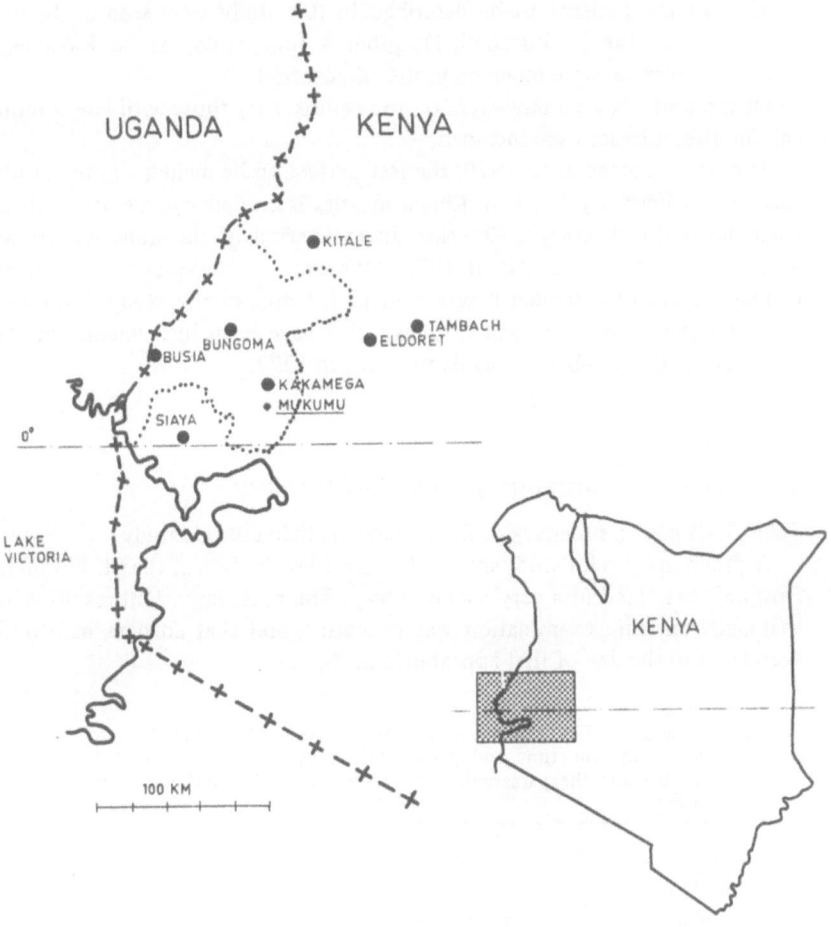

Map 3.1. Western Province, Kenya and some nearby district headquarters. Western Province and Siaya District were regularly visited on safaris by the Mobile Eye Unit no. 5. The other places were more or less frequently visited by the ophthalmologist alone, for consultations. The asterix indicates the location of the St. Elizabeth Hospital Mukumu

Kakamega. The eye department (founded and run by the Professor Weve Foundation) has at its disposal a 28 bed in-patient facility and a large out-patient department.

The "Kenya Society for the Blind" runs a nationwide, therapeutic, mobile eye service, and one of their "Mobile Eye Unit" 's has its home base at this hospital. With the Mobile Eye Unit, regular safaris were made in Western Province and the Siaya District, which together covers an area with over 2 million inhabitants. Most of the routine work on these safaris was done by the Ophthalmic Clinical Officer, and his assistants: a driver and a dresser.

Most of the patients to be described in this study were seen in the isolation ward of the St. Elizabeth Hospital. A few patients at the Kakamega Provincial Hospital were included in the clinical trial.

Of the patients seen anywhere on our safaris, only those with late complications after measles were included.

The study started June 1975; the last patient to be included in this study was seen in February 1978. In Kenya measles is an endemic disease, with an epidemic outbreak every 2–3 years. In the period of the study we had an epidemic in the second half of 1976. Moreover, in November 1976 a large measles vaccination campaign was held in the area of this study, a total of 18,000 doses were given and this may also have been instrumental in the reduction of the number of measles patients in 1977.

3.2. The patients

Groups of patients: diagnosis of measles and treatment

Table 3.2.a gives a summary of the patients included in this study.

A preliminary pilot study involved 99 measles children at the St. Elizabeth Hospital, examined in a very irregular way. The most important results were that daily slitlamp examination was necessary, and that all data had to be correlated to the day of first appearance of the rash.

Table 3.2.a. The different groups of measles patients, included into this study, the time and place where they were examined, their number and the paragraph where their clinical description is to be found.

	Time	Place	No.	Description
Pilot Study	6-'75–4-'76	SEH	99	
Mukumu I	6-'76–11-'76	SEH	148	§ 4.1-4.2
Clinical trial	3-'77–10-'77			
Mukumu II		SEH	51	
Kakamega		KPH	49	§ 4.3.2
Safaris + Mukumu	1-'77–2-'78	any	9	§ 4.4

SEH = St. Elizabeth Hospital; KPH = Kakamega Provincial Hospital.

In this study four groups of patients will be described. The most important group is "Mukumu I" including 148 patients seen at the time of the measles epidemic in 1976. These patients will be described in detail in §4.1.

The statistical analysis regarding measles keratitis and nutritional status is done on this group only. For statistical reasons it is not possible to combine the different groups of our patients.

The 100 patients in the groups "Mukumu II" and "Kakamega" formed a clinical trial regarding the effectiveness of Vitamin A capsules 200,000 IU and (or) tetracycline eye-ointment, in the prevention of corneal complications in measles. This trial failed because of the limited number of patients. Only the patients who developed complications will be described.

During the safaris I used to check on all children admitted to the hospitals and dispensaries we visited. This means that every year about 2,000 children were examined, apart from those seen at the regular eye clinics. In 1977, 7 patients with late complications after measles were found on safaris. They are included in §4.4.

Diagnosis of measles

All children seen at the out-patients department with measles were admitted, except when the mother refused admission. I did not interfere actively with this policy. The diagnosis of measles was made on clinical grounds by the attending (pediatric) clinical officer or physician and this clinical diagnosis was, ipso facto, the reason for admission to the isolation ward and inclusion into this study.

The demonstration of a specific IgM is proof of a recent infection (Wilterdink 1979). A total of 118 serum samples were examined for the presence of anti-measles IgM; 106 were positive, 12 negative.

The 12 patients with negative IgM estimations are tabulated in table 3.2.b.

Table 3.2.b. Patients with negative anti-measles IgM in relation to the time of outbreak of the rash (R), nutritional status (W/A = Weight for Age), the keratitis classification (§ 3.3), vaccination against measles and the tentative explanation for the negative IgM.

R	W/A	Keratitis classification	Measles vaccination	Tentative explanation
− 1	64	II	+	too early
− 1	81	III	−	too early
0	87	neg	−	too early
0	76	II	−	too early
0		I	−	too early
+ 1	maln.	V	−	malnutrition
+ 2	66	III	−	malnutrition
+ 2	93	III	−	?
+ 3	90	neg	−	no measles
+ 4	86	neg	−	no measles
+ 6	58	I	?	no measles/maln.
+ 7	76	V	−	?

In 5 cases the sample was probably taken too early, i.e. before or on the day of the outbreak of the rash. In 2 or 3 cases the possibility of immuno-suppression or delay in the development of measles-antibodies, due to Protein Energy Malnutrition, exists, whereas in 2 or 3 other cases the eruption might have been something other than measles. For 2 cases no explanation can be given. This outcome once more proves the validity of the clinical diagnosis of measles (Gemert et al. 1977) and makes it more than likely — especially in epidemics — that we really are dealing with measles patients.

Sex, age and time of admission. (Mukumu I)

During the epidemic of 1976, 152 children, all Luhya's by tribe, were admitted to the isolation ward of the St. Elizabeth Hospital. Three children were excluded from this study, because they had developed measles more than 10 days previously. One well-nourished child with a measles contact failed to develop a measles rash and was therefore also excluded from the study.

The remaining 148 children were 78 girls and 68 boys; in 2 cases the sex was not recorded (for numerical data, see appendix). The age of these children varied from 5 months to 14 years, median age 21 months. The age distribution is given in table 3.2.c.

The time of admission in relation to the day of outbreak of the rash is given in table 3.2.d.

The conclusion to be drawn from tables 3.2.c and 3.2.d is that our measles patients are, as is usually seen in Africa, quite young when they contract measles. Moreover, they are admitted to the hospital early after the outbreak of the rash, probably because the mothers recognize the seriousness of the disease.

Treatment of measles patients

From the beginning of the study it was decided not to interfere with the treatment as prescribed by the attending clinical officer or physician.

All children received antibiotics (mostly penicilline) and anti-malaria

Table 3.2.c. Age of measles patients included in Mukumu I (median age 21 months).

Age in months	0–12	13–24	25–36	37–48	49 +	Total
Number of patients	30	49	31	18	20	148

Table 3.2.d. The day of admission of the 148 measles patients in Mukumu I in relation to the day of outbreak of the rash.

Day of admission	− 3	− 2	− 1	R	1	2	3	4	5 +	Total
Number of patients	1	–	3	17	58	26	22	14	7	148

treatment systemically. Fluids were given in large quantities, when necessary in intravenous-drips or subcutaneously. Phenergan syrup or other cough mixtures and nasal drops were given for symptomatic relief. The oral ulcers were painted with gentian violet. Occasionally children needed to be nursed in steam tents. The treatment also included the administration – routinely – of extra vitamins, in relatively low dosage. The children daily received an average of about 1,000 IU Vit A extra (together with B1, B2, B6, B12, C, nicotinamide, Ca Panthotenate). When the condition of the children permitted the intake of solid food, they had the customary posho (maize) with mboga (green leafy vegetable).

Out of the 148 children in the "Mukumu I" group 11 children died.

In 84 cases the attending clinical officer (or doctor) prescribed tetracycline eye-ointment, because of the conspicuously red aspect of the eyes. This treatment was accepted and handled as a clinical trial as to the effect of tetracycline eye-ointment on the keratitis. We only interfered with this regimen when ocular complications developed.

3.3. Ophthalmological examination

The ophthalmological examination consisted of a daily examination with a hand held slitlamp (KOWA). Vital stains were used to enhance the visibility of the epithelial lesions: fluorescein 1% was used for the lesions of the cornea, Rose Bengal 1% (colour index 45440) (RB) and, later on, Lissamine Green 1% (colour index 44090) (LG) were used to stain the lesions of the conjunctival epithelium.

A lot of confusion exists about the etiological interpretation of the staining conjunctival lesions. According to Norn (1970, 1973) RB and LG stain degenerating and dead cells in the epithelium, irrespective of the cause of the lesions. On the contrary Sauter (1976) claims that "– vital staining by 1% Rose Bengal or 1% Lissamine Green is a *safe, sensitive, specific, simple* and *cheap* method for – early – detection of cases of conjunctival xerosis (X-1A), both in Health Centres and in large-scale field surveys." (pg 194). This claim could not be confirmed (Kusin, Soewondo and Parlindungan Sinaga, 1979; Sommer, 1980).

The use of the word "specific" is the cause of this controversy. For the subject of this study it is of critical importance how the staining conjunctival lesions are etiologically interpreted. Why I adhere to Norn's opinion, will be explained in §3.4.

In contrast to RB and LG, fluorescein stains "spaces": when an epithelial defect exists, fluorescein diffuses into the intercellular spaces (Norn 1970). Fig. 3.3. (see colour plate I) gives a good example of this differential staining in a case of herpetic keratitis. (= Pat Chw P 172, §4.4.)

In the examination of the cornea a quantitative scoring system was used to evaluate the correlation measles-keratitis and nutritional status. The number of lesions on the cornea was counted. If no lesions were present, this was considered negative, 1--5 lesions was positive, 6 lesions or more + +. The observations of both corneae during the first 5 consecutive days were totalled. The maximum to be reached was therefore 20 +. The "keratitis score" was classified as follows:

extent and duration of corneal lesions	classes of keratitis score
0 +	I
1 and 2 +	II
3–5 +	III
6–8 +	IV
9–20+	V

When in the first 5 days, one observation day was missing, an interpolation between the previous and following day was used. No "keratitis score" was calculated when the period of observation had been less than 5 days. In some tables a "negative" keratitis score is mentioned instead of a keratitis score class I. This means that the observation period was less than 5 days and for that reason — by definition — no classification of keratitis score could be made.

The ophthalmological examination was — because of the purpose of the study and the generally bad condition of the children — limited to a slitlamp examination. No attention was given to the posterior segment of the eye.

The nearest microbiological laboratory from which reliable results could be obtained was some hundreds of kilometers away. To culture viruses or bacteria was therefore not possible.

3.4. The significance of vital staining of the conjunctiva with Lissamine Green or Rose Bengal

Lack of specificity for the detection of Vitamin A deficiency

Rose Bengal (Colour Index 45440) and Lissamine Green (Colour Index 44090) are in a 1% solution in use for the examination of the conjunctival epithelium. Lissamine Green has the advantage over Rose Bengal of a better visibility against a reddish background and hurts less on instillation. They stain mucus and devitalized cells, irrespective of the cause of the cellular damage (Passmore & King 1955; Norn 1970, 1973). The positive staining with Rose Bengal and Lissamine Green nearly always (except, among others, in measles) takes the form of micropunctate lesions. When present in small numbers, they have no pathological significance (Kronning 1954; Norn 1964, 1970, 1973; Lansche 1965). They occur in pathological quantities in kerato-conjunctivitis sicca (M. Sjögren) (Kronning 1954; Passmore & King 1955), in traumata of the conjunctival epithelium (mechanical or toxic), sometimes around Bitot's spots. In 1976 Sauter claimed that a positive staining with Rose Bengal and Lissamine Green was a specific and reliable sign of Vitamin A deficiency. This claim has not been confirmed.

Vijayaraghavan et al. (1978) studied under field conditions the usefulness of the Rose Bengal test for the detection of Vitamin A deficiency. They found a considerable number of false positive children: i.e. children who are positive in the dye test, but fail to show any -- clinical or biochemical -- sign of Vitamin A deficiency.

Kusin et al. (1977) demonstrated the presence of a considerable number of false negatives. Moreover, in a clinical trial, the treatment with a massive dose of Vitamin A (200,000 iU) failed to protect the children against the subsequent development of a positive dye test (Kusin, Soewondo and Parlindungan Sinaga 1979). These findings were confirmed by Sommer (1980) and he reaches the conclusion that the staining with Lissamine Green is useless in the detection of Vitamin A deficiency.

All this work has been done in Asia (India and Indonesia). Unaware of this work, I paid a lot of attention to the value of Lissamine Green test in its relation to Vitamin A deficiency. Early 1976 I did a survey in the Shikusa Borstal Institution, Kenya, where among the inmates clinical signs of Vitamin A deficiency were rather frequent. In a statistical analysis (W. Gemert, Medical Research Centre, Nairobi, Dpt. of the Royal Tropical Institute, Amsterdam, The Netherlands) it was found that the incidence of Bitot's spots correlated significantly with the time spent in prison. No such correlation existed between the Lissamine Green staining alone (i.e. without the presence of Bitot's spots) and the length of stay in prison (see table 3.4.a.).

Also a doubly masked clinical trial was done. Half the inmates got 200,000 iU Vitamin A, the other a placebo. After one month all inmates were re-examined for the presence of clinical signs of Vitamin A deficiency and the Lissamine Green test. The results are given in table 3.4.b.

It appeared that 20% of all boys, who had been negative for L.G. at the initial survey, became positive, whether they got Vitamin A or a placebo. Also, 18% of the boys, initially positive, became negative after the placebo, whereas 37% became negative after Vitamin A. This difference is statistically significant. The only conclusion can be that some epithelial lesions staining with Lissamine Green react to the administration of Vitamin A.

Because of these results I reached the conclusion that Lissamine Green is not a test for Vitamin A deficiency which later was confirmed by others.

Lissamine Green in measles

Around the outbreak of the rash Lissamine Green and Rose Bengal staining lesions were observed in the bulbar conjunctiva (§ 4.1.2, figs. 4.1.2.a and b). They had a particular morphology, quite different from the micropunctate lesions around Bitot's spots and in xerosis. They disappeared without any

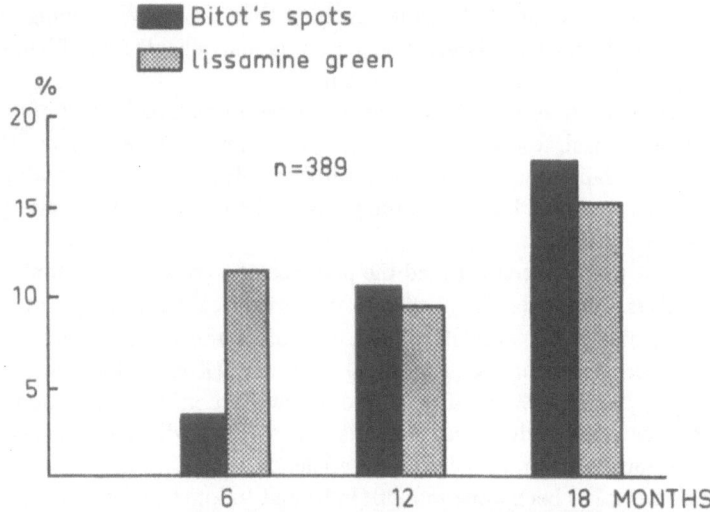

Table 3.4.a. The incidence of Bitot's spots and Lissamine Green positive staining, in relation to the time spent in the Borstal Institution. The incidence of Bitot's spots and the duration of the stay are significantly correlated, no association exists between the time spent in prison and the incidence of Lissamine Green positive staining.

treatment and were seen in *all* patients who came under observation before the outbreak of the rash (table 4.1.2.c).

Moreover, the studies mentioned earlier in this section don't substantiate

Table 3.4.b. The staining with Lissamine Green before and after the treatment with Vitamin or a placebo. The administration of a high dose of Vitamin A reduces significantly (compared to placebo) the incidence of Lissamine Green positive staining (compare Groups A and C, $P = 0.015$). The administration of Vitamin A does not prevent the conversion from negative to positive staining in 20% of pupils (compare Groups B and D, $P = 0.40$). At least a very considerable proportion of the Lissamine Green staining appears therefore to be independent of the Vitamin A status.

Staining at initial survey	Staining at control survey	
	After Vitamin A	
	LG +	LG −
Group A: LG +	63%	37%
Group B: LG −	20%	80%
Group C: LG +	79%	21%
Group D: LG −·	18%	82%
	LG +	LG −
	After placebo	

n = 389

the specificity, claimed by Sauter, for Lissamine Green to detect conjunctival xerosis.

For these two reasons, the peculiar morphology and natural history of the conjunctival lesions in measles, and the lack of etiological specificity for Lissamine Green there are no grounds to follow Sauter's opinion that these lesions are specifically caused by Vitamin A deficiency.

In this study LG and RB will therefore only be considered as vital stains for the detection of epithelial lesions, without ascribing any precise etiological connotation, unless proven by other techniques.

In §5.1 it will be demonstrated that with the use of immunofluorescent techniques these lesions reveal their viral nature.

3.5. Assessment of the nutritional status

When the nutritional status of a measles child is to be compared with the severity of its measles keratitis, the nutritional status of the child must be measured quantitatively: a qualitative clinical impression is useless for this purpose, so anthropometric or biochemical methods are to be used.

On admission, the nurses of the isolation wards collected data regarding age, sex, vaccinations and measles-contacts of the children. As soon as feasible the nurses took height and weight of the admitted children. Height was taken with the children lying on the bed, using an ordinary tape ruler; weight was taken with ordinary baby weighing scales. The sometimes critical condition of the children and the application of drips and steam-tents did not permit the use of Salter scales. Occasionally measuring was, in any event, impossible.

Weight, height and age, are, in any combination, used to asses the nutritional status.
— Weight for age (W/A): the weight is expressed as a percentage of the ideal weight for the age of the child. Although it is an American standard, the Harvard standard is generally used as reference. The "Road to Health" is based on this standard. (Ministry of Health, Kenyan Government.)
— Height for Age (H/A): the height is expressed as a percentage of the ideal height for the age of the child. Stunting would be indicative of malnutrition of long duration.
— Weight for Height (W/H): the weight is expressed as a percentage of the ideal weight for the height of the child. This index is extremely useful when the age of the child is not exactly known. Moreover, it would be a good indicator of the actual nutritional status of the child (Alleyne et al. 1977).

Height, weight and age can mathematically be combined in single indices, which are then supposed to be independant of the age of the child (Rao and Singh 1970; Dugdale 1971; McLaren and Read 1975). They are, however, only applicable to a limited age group (up to 5 years), moreover, our data were not always complete enough to use these indices.

To evaluate the nutritional status biochemically, as soon as possible after admission, a venous bloodsample was drawn, spun down, and the serum was stored at $-20°C$. These samples were transported to the Medical Research Centre (Nairobi), where all immunological and biochemical estimations were done (Miss H.L. Ensering and Miss M.M. van Rens).

For the detection of specific anti-measles IgM a direct immunofluorescent technique was used. Vero cells (Green monkey kidney cells), in tubes with coverslips were inoculated with the Schwarz measles vaccine strain. When, during inoculation at 37°, a Cyto-Pathogene Effect, typical for measles, appeared, these coverslips were washed three times with Phosphate Buffered Saline (PBS), and fixed in acetone for 20 minutes at a temperature of minus 20°C and kept at 4°C. Three coverslips were inoculated simultaneously with either the serum to be examined, diluted 1:10 in PBS, or a standard IgM positive serum or a standard IgM negative serum, but with specific anti-measles IgG.

After incubation at 37°C for 45 minutes and washing three times with PBS, the Fluorescein-Iso-Thiocyanate-Conjugate (FITC)-anti-human-Igm-goat-serum was applied. After incubation and washing with PBS the coverslips were mounted and checked for the presence of fluorescence under the fluorescence microscope. Only a strong fluorescence was read as positive.

The results of the 118 anti-measles IgM estimations are given in § 3.2.

99 Serum samples were estimated for the presence of serum retinol and β carotene. The values found were far too high to be reliable, which was probably caused by autofluorescence because of improper storage. These results will therefore not be used.

In 103 sera RBP was estimated, the albumin content in 100 samples. For both estimations a Manchini Radial Immuno-Diffusion Test was used.

Glassplates, $100 \times 100 \times 1.5$ mm, were coated with 1% Agar Noble and dried for 15 min at 100°C. A solution of 2% agarose in Manchini-buffer was mixed with commercially available antiserum (Hoechst) at 53°C: 0.8 cc of anti-Retinol-Binding-Protein serum, or 0.3 cc of anti-albumin-serum was added to 15 cc of the agarose solution. This mixture was poured out on the glassplates, 2.5 mm large holes were punched in this gel with a gel-puncher. Each hole was filled with 5 μl, either of a standard serum in routine-dilutions, or the serum to be tested in a 1:150 dilution.

The plates were left (strictly horizontally) for 2–3 days in which the proteins diffused into the agarose-gel, where they precipitated with the specific antiproteins. The size of the precipitation-ring is a measure for the quantity of protein present in the serum to be tested. The value can be calculated by comparison with the precipitation rings of the standard serum.

In this technique, the normal values (derived from Europeans) are:

Albumin: 3500–5500 mgr%

Retinol Binding Protein: 3–6 mgr%

The results will be presented in § 6.2.

3.6. Biopsies and specimens for pathology, electronmicroscopy and immunofluorescence

After consent of the attending parent was obtained, paired conjunctival biopsies were taken from 10 children: one biopsy came from the Lissamine Green positive area in the exposed part of the bulbar conjunctiva, one biopsy — serving as a control — from the non-staining conjunctival tarsi.

For conjunctival biopsies, the conjunctiva was anaesthetized with a few drops of 0.4% descaine (Novesine ®) topically. The conjunctiva was lifted with a non-toothed forceps and a small piece was cut off with a sterile de Wecker scissor. For obvious reasons it was not possible to obtain corneal biopsies.

Four pairs of conjunctival biopsies were fixed in glutaraldehyde according to Sabatini, and prepared for electronmicroscopy (Drs. G.F.J.M. Vrensen and J.J.L. van der Want) at the Netherlands Ophthalmic Research Institute, Amsterdam.

Five pairs of conjunctival biopsies were taken from children admitted to the measles-ward of the Kenyatta National Hospital (Head of the department Dr. M.L. Oduori), and — stored in B.M. Eagles with 2% Foetal Bovine Serum — airmailed on dry ice to Dr. F.E. Nommensen (Dpt. of Virology, Erasmus University, Rotterdam) for investigation with immunofluorescent techniques.

One pair of conjunctival biopsies was taken from a measles child with conjunctival xerosis and prepared for light microscopy.

One child, with a corneal necrosis after measles, came for evisceration of the affected eye. One corneal specimen was sent to Prof. Dr. W.A. Manschot, Inst. of Pathology, Erasmus University, Rotterdam; a second specimen was examined by electron-microscopy.

In 2 children who developed complications (one central abrasion and one an ulcer) and died, we were allowed to remove the corneae. They were sent for electronmicroscopy.

3.7. Representativeness of the patient samples

In this study nearly all the children examined were hospitalized. This might easily become an important cause for selection of the patients to be examined:

(a) Only the more malnourished children are seen, because they are supposedly more susceptible to infections and, in the case of malnutrition, infections run a more severe course.

(b) The admission of children to a hospital is always to be paid for. For this purpose a government hospital is much cheaper than a Mission hospital. It is therefore quite conceivable, that in the St. Elizabeth Hospital only children of more well-to-do families are admitted and hence these children might be in a better nutritional state than the average population.

Table 3.7.a. The percentage of children, age 13–48 months, below the indicated level of Weight for Age. The first group is a random sample survey of 229 children, included in the Rural Kenyan Nutrition Survey (1977). The second group are the 72 children, age 13–48 months of the measles patients in Mukumu I. In the column with 'weight correction' the weightloss because of measles (6%: Morley, Woodland and Martin 1963) has been taken into account.

| Weight for Age | Rural Kenyan Nutrition Survey | Measles patients | |
| | | Weight correction | |
		yes	no
< 70%	2%	0%	3%
< 80%	7%	10%	14%
< 90%	27%	26%	46%
	n = 229	n = 72	

Table 3.7.b. Comparison of Height for Age of 229 children, age 13–48 months, seen in the Rural Kenyan Nutrition Survey and the 73 measles patients, age 13–48 months, in measles patients group Mukumu I.

Height for Age	Rural Kenyan Nutrition Survey	Measles patients
< 80%	2%	1%
< 90%	21%	26%
	n = 229	n = 73

Table 3.7.c. Comparison of the Weight for Age of the children, seen in the Provincial Hospital Kakamega, and the St. Elizabeth Hospital Mukuma, during 1977. No statistically significant differences were present.

| | Weight for Age | | | |
	< 60%	60–80%	> 80%	
Kakamega	1	22	22	45
Mukumu I	3	21	21	45
	4	43	43	90

ad (a) In 1977, the Kenyan Ministry of Finance and Planning published the results from the "Rural Kenyan Nutrition Survey". Table 3.7.a shows that the 148 children in the most important group of our patients (Mukumu I) are a representative sample of the children in Western Province as far as their Weight for Age is concerned.

The similarity is especially good when the fact is taken into account that children with measles loose weight, because of measles. In West Africa an average weightloss of 6% was found

(Morley, Woodland and Martin 1963) and in the column with "weight correction" this figure is used.

Table 3.7.b shows the concordance for Height for Age in our patients and the sample of the Rural Kenyan Nutrition Survey.

ad (b) Table 3.7.c shows a comparison of the Weight for Age of the children in the Provincial Hospital Kakamega and the children in the St. Elizabeth Hospital. The numbers are small, but in our material, the suggestion that children in the St. Elizabeth Hospital are in a better nutritional status, compared to the children in the Governmental Hospital, cannot be substantiated.

This leads to the conclusion that our measles patients form a group of children representative for those in Western Province.

4 – Clinical description of Ocular signs and Corneal complications of Measles

4.1. Ocular involvement in measles

The clinical description of the ocular lesions in measles is derived from the daily slitlamp-examination of the 148 children in "Mukumu I", during the measles epidemic in 1976. In the well-known catarrhal conjunctivitis of prodromal measles a distinction could be made into two different disease-entities: a subepithelial conjunctivitis and an epithelial conjunctivokeratitis. The former occurs early and is localized in the subepithelial tissue, mainly of the tarsal, and less of the bulbar, conjunctiva, whereas the latter occurs some days later, is strictly epithelial and is localized in the exposed parts of the bulbar conjunctiva.

4.1.1. Subepithelial conjunctivitis

A catarrhal conjunctivitis was a constant, but in extent variable, feature of the prodromal and early exanthematous stage of measles.

The palpebral conjunctiva was always inflamed, and in at least half of the cases an inflammatory reaction of also the bulbar conjunctiva was conspicuous without separating the eyelids. The discharge varied from watery to, later on, mucoid. A sometimes frankly purulent discharge suggested bacterial involvement. In some cases a slight oedema of the conjunctiva at the inner canthus existed, subsiding within a few days. No lesions comparable to Koplik's spots were observed in the conjunctiva.

5–7 Days after the outbreak of the rash this conjunctivitis had disappeared. Subconjunctival haemorrhages occured in some 20% of the cases. Follicles were visible in the lower fornix or at the border of the superior tarsal plate in 10–20% of the cases.

4.1.2. Epithelial conjunctivokeratitis

Conjunctiva

With the use of Lissamine Green or Rose Bengal the presence of epithelial lesions in the conjunctiva could be demonstrated. These lesions were otherwise not visible. They were localized at the nasal part of the bulbar conjunctiva, a little less frequently at the temporal side, but nearly always in the exposed parts of the conjunctiva in the interpalpebral fissure (fig. 4.1.2a: see colour plate II). Only in 3 (of the 148) cases were these lesions observed at the palpebral conjunctiva. In these cases also their number was very limited.

The shape of these lesions varied a great deal. Usually they were more or less round, but occasionally they were multi-angular, circular or horse-shoe shaped (fig. 4.1.2.b: see colour plate II), their size varied from 0.2–0.4 mm.

The number of these "measles spots" varied considerably. On some

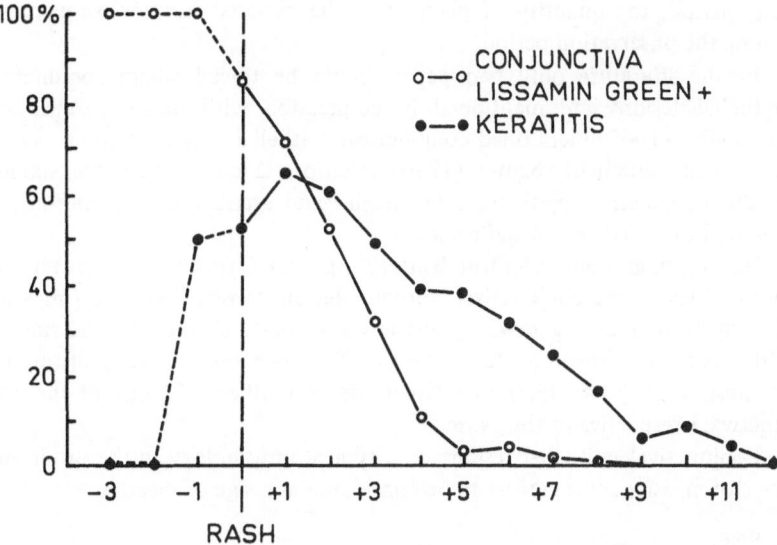

Figure 4.1.2.c. The incidence of Lissamine Green staining conjunctival epithelial lesions and keratitis, in relation to the day of outbreak of the rash (R). The data before R are drawn with interrupted lines to indicate the lower level of reliability (compared to data after R) because of the limited number of observations of these early cases

occasions only a single spot was present, whereas in other cases they could be numerous and give the impression to conflate to a single, large, intensely staining area on the conjunctiva.

The presence of the "measles spots" was dependent on the stage of the disease. All 6 children examined in the prodromal stage of the measles showed these lesions. From the day of the outbreak of the rash the incidence of these lesions dropped, to reach a level of only 11% at the fourth day after the rash. No "measles spots" were seen in the conjunctiva after the eighth day (fig. 4.1.2.c).

These "measles spots" were present independently of the presence of sub-epithelial vasodilatation.

The "measles spots" had a life-span of one to only a few days and disappeared spontaneously without any treatment. The conjunctival epithelium with "measles spots" is usually not water-repellent: conjunctival xerosis was only observed in 4 cases; two times a capsule of Vitamin A (200.000 iU) was given, the 2 other children received no treatment. In all four patients the conjunctivae returned to normal within a few days.

The shape, the distribution, and the size of these lesions is characteristic for measles; their appearance differs from other conditions in which staining of the conjunctival epithelium occurs. I never observed them in diseases other than measles.

The impression exists that in some children who could be observed for a long period, the quantity of pigment in the exposed conjunctiva increased during the observation period.

In the literature only two papers could be traced where conjunctival epithelial lesions are mentioned in connection with measles. Azizi and Krakovsky (1965) mentioned conjunctival epithelial lesions, without elaborating their statement. Sauter (1976) mentions a coarse punctate staining of the conjunctival epithelium in measles and ascribes this finding not to measles but to Vitamin A deficiency.

Our findings don't confirm Sauter's opinion (cfr §3.4). Moreover, the morphology of the conjunctival epithelial lesions is very typical for measles. This in itself is an argument against any specificity claimed for the staining with Lissamine Green or Rose Bengal. This fact once more confirms the conclusion of §3.4: Lissamine Green stains epithelial lesions of the conjunctiva, irrespective of the cause.

Conjunctival epithelial lesions of a typical morphology in the prodromal stage of measles are therefore to be considered as a sign of measles.

Cornea

Usually the "measles spots" in the conjunctival epithelium had their largest extent around the day of outbreak of the rash (R). Sometimes the whole of the nasal and temporal exposed conjunctiva stained brilliantly green. The lesions did not stay restricted to the conjunctival epithelium, but the same lesions developed at the corneal side of the limbus, in continuity with the lesions in the conjunctival epithelium (fig. 4.1.2.d: see colour plate II).

The epithelial conjunctivitis crosses over to the cornea to give a coarse punctate keratitis. In one case, where I had taken a biopsy from the conjunctiva, only the part of the cornea adjacent to the site of the biopsy stayed free from the keratitis. This confirms the clinical impression that the measles keratitis develops from the epithelial conjunctivitis.

The appearance in size and shape of the lesions in the conjunctival and corneal epithelium was identical. In the cornea the lesions were visible without vital staining. Here they appeared as greyish, slightly opaque, epithelial lesions, strictly confined to the epithelium: Bowman's membrane and the stroma were not involved.

The epithelial keratitis progressed from the limbus toward the centre of the cornea (fig. 4.1.2.e: see colour plate II).

At the time when the conjunctival epithelial lesions started to disappear, the corneal epithelium at the limbus also began to regain its normal aspect. The superficial, coarse punctate keratitis now occupied the mid-periphery of the corneal epithelium (fig. 4.1.2.f: see colour plate II). The centre of the cornea was the last part to become involved. In many cases a punctate keratitis centrally in the cornea was the last manifestation of this measles conjunctivo-keratitis (fig. 4.1.2.g: see colour plate II).

This conjunctivo-keratitis was sometimes observed in restricted forms.

Several times the keratitis stopped at the corneal side of the limbus and did not progress towards the centre. On other occasions only a limited number of lesions were observed, and only one or a few spots developed during a 10 day observation. The time of appearance of the lesions is variable, not the sequence. The limbal lesions appeared from $R - 1$ to $R + 5$, the central lesions from $R + 2$ to $R + 9$ to 11. R (like elsewhere in this study) indicates here the day of outbreak of the rash. No lesions were seen after day $R + 11$.

The keratitis heals without sequelae. In 7 of the 248 cases however, macro-erosions were seen, directly attributable to the keratitis. They will be dealt with in the next paragraph. No significant differences were observed between right and left eyes.

This keratitis was observed in 115 of the 148 patients (76%). In fig. 4.1.2.c also the incidence of this measles-keratitis is given in relation to the day of outbreak of the rash (R). The incidence is highest at day $R + 1$: 65% of the measles children show at that day a keratitis. From that day onwards the incidence decreases. No keratitis was observed after day $R + 11$.

Comparison of the graphs in fig. 4.1.2.c shows that the conjunctival epithelial lesions occur earlier than the corneal lesions, as was to be expected from the clinical description.

The finding that the incidence of the keratitis is lower than the incidence of the conjunctival epithelial lesions, and the observation that even an extensive measles keratitis at the corneal side of the limbus can be stopped there, suggests the existence of a kind of protective mechanism.

Probably the development of neutralizing antibodies is the cause of this phenomenon, it is, however, not possible to answer this question from the available data.

4.2. "Exaggerated signs" and early corneal complications

In the previous paragraph the ocular signs of measles in 148 measles patients were described. A distinction was made between a prodromal subepithelial conjunctivitis and a strictly epithelial conjunctivo-keratitis. Both are signs of measles.

In this paragraph the early corneal sequelae, exceeding the normal keratitis, occurring during the initial stay in the hospital will be described. Out of the 248 children, seen daily in the Provincial Hospital, Kakamega and the St Elizabeth Hospital, Mukumu, 7 developed macro-erosions of the cornea. The pathogenesis of these macro-erosions is essentially the same as for the smaller lesions of the measles-keratitis. Their "exaggerated" size might quite well be relevant for the purpose of this study. For this reason they are described here separately and more extensively.

3 out of the 248 children developed exposure ulcers because of the inability to close their eyes. An exposure ulcer is to be considered as a real, early corneal complication of measles.

In the pilot study and in safari patients the same phenomena were observed: 5 macro-erosions and 2 exposure ulcers. These will not be described here.

Those complications to be described in §4.4 are considered late complications, when they developed after the acute stage of measles, but within a time span of 3 months after the rash. The period of 3 months was chosen arbitrarily to be to some extent sure of the relationship with measles. Late complications were less frequently seen than the early ones. They are far more difficult to trace: the mortality in complicated cases of measles is higher, and in the bush medical help is seldom searched for. The restriction that the complication had to be seen within 3 months after the rash greatly reduced the number of patients with late complications (9) who could be included in this study.

No late or severe ocular complications were seen in the 248 children in Kakamega and Mukumu, and no permanent ocular damage was observed in these children, apart from a single patient with minimal corneal nebulae.

4.2.1. Central corneal macro-erosions

7 out of the 248 patients − 4 boys and 3 girls − developed a central corneal erosion: in the central part of the cornea the epithelium was shed, without involvement of Bowman's membrane or the stromal tissue. The limbus always stayed free. Fig. 4.2.1.a (see colour plate III) is a good example of a corneal erosion after measles.

In 3 cases the erosions were bilateral, in 4 cases only one eye was affected. The erosions developed at day $R + 1$, $R + 1$, $R + 1$, $R + 1$, $R + 8$, $R + 8$ and $R + 9$.

In some cases the erosions developed in an area of active measles-keratitis, of which the patient presented in Fig. 4.2.1.b (see colour plate III) and c is a good example.

The treatment consisted of tetracyclin 1% eye ointment topically, along with padding of the affected eye(s). The children also had a capsule of 200,000 iU Vitamin A. The erosions healed within 1−5 days.

Especially in some safari-patients it was observed that the corneal erosion was localized in the exposed part of the cornea: some children were so debilitated that closure of the eyelids became a problem. Probably this is a transition to the exposure ulcers to be described in the next paragraph.

Patient M 245 (fig. 4.2.1.d.) is an example of such an erosion.

This 9 months old girl developed a corneal erosion at the six o'clock position on the first day after outbreak of the rash. She was treated with tetracycline eye-ointment, 6−10 times daily. The ever-present mother was instructed to keep the eyelids closed. No pad and bandage were applied, because of the extremely bad condition of the child. She also had a capsule of 200,000 iU Vitamin A. The cornea healed within 3 days without sequelae.

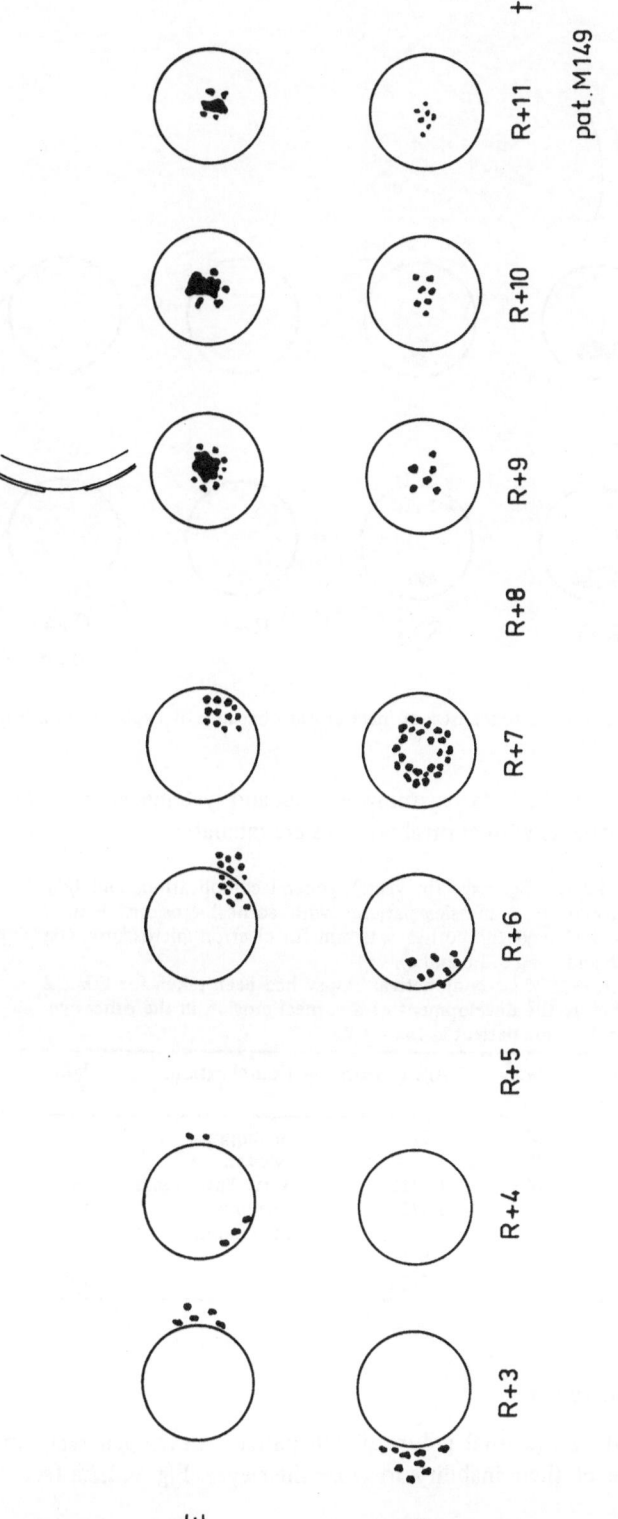

Figure 4.2.1.c. The same patients (M 149) as fig. 4.2.1.b. The course of the measles keratitis and the subsequent corneal erosion is given here in full detail. The cornea was sent for electronmicroscopy (fig. 5.3.b and c)

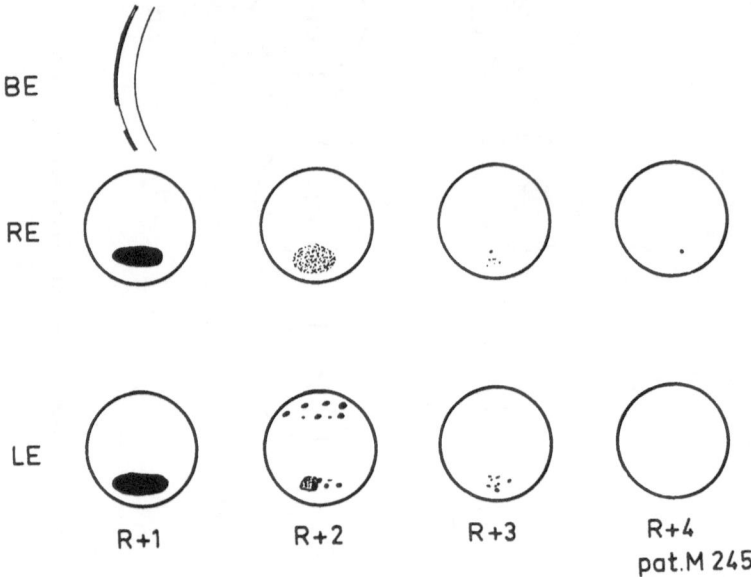

Figure 4.2.1.d. The occurrence of a corneal erosion because of exposure in a 9 month old girl with measles

In table 4.2.1.e. the data regarding age, sex and systemic complications of the 7 measles patients with corneal erosions are tabulated.

Table 4.2.1.e. Sex, age (in years), general complications and IgM estimations in 7 measles patients with corneal erosions. Patient M 149 died, and the cornea was sent for electron-microscopy. (fig 4.2.1 b and c, fig 5.3 b and c).
In patient M 223 a conjunctival biopsy had been taken for E.M., 2 days before the development of a corneal erosion in the other eye. This is the same patient as fig. 4.1.2.e.

Patients number	Sex	Age in years	Complications	IgM
M 61	M	1.2/12	Meningitis	+
M 113	F	3	Pneumonia	+
M 149	M	1.6/12	Virus Pneumonia	—
M 223	M	1.9/12	Pneumonia	nd
M 241	M	7/12	Pneumonia	—
M 245	F	9/12	—	nd
K 19	F	2.2/12	—	nd

nd = not done

4.2.2. Exposure ulcers

3 children out of the total group of 248 patients developed real exposure ulcers because of their inability to close their eyes. Fig. 4.2.2.a (see colour

Table 4.2.2.c. The sex, age, general complications and IgM estimation in 3 patients with exposure of the cornea. Patients M 7 and M 207 died. The cornea of patient M 207 was available for microscropic examination.

Patients number	Sex	Age in years	Complications	IgM
M 7	M	4	Malnutrition + TB Meningitis	+ later on –
M 117	M	5	–	+
M 207	M	2 6/12	Dehydration Malnutrition	nd

nd = not done

plate III) shows a typical example of such an exposure ulcer. Pat M 7, a 4 year old boy developed exposure-erosions, 3 days after outbreak of the rash, in both eyes. These erosions reacted favourably to treatment. Three weeks later an exposure ulcer suddenly appeared in the right eye. The next morning the boy died.

A $2\frac{1}{2}$ year old boy was admitted, 9 days after the outbreak of the rash, with an exposure ulcer at the six o'clock position in his right eye. The next morning the boy died. The cornea was available for study under the electron-microscope.

Pat M 117, a 5 year old boy, developed a typical exposure at day R + 5, four days after his admission. In fig. 4.2.2.b the clinical course of his exposure ulcers is depicted in more detail. The corneae healed within 5 days with the development of corneal nebulae.

The data regarding age, sex, IgM estimations and systemic complications are given in table 4.2.2.c.

When the patients with the corneal macro-erosions are compared with the patients with exposure ulcers, clinically two differences are apparent:

(a) The patients with corneal erosions have or had a more severe measles-keratitis than the children with exposure ulcers.

(b) The children with exposure ulcers were generally more ill than the children with the central erosions.

These observations suggest that the corneal erosions are a direct progression of the measles-keratitis. This view is confirmed by the findings in the electron-microscope. (§5.3).

On the other hand, the exposure ulcers appear to be more correlated with the severity of the systemic disease than with the measles-keratitis.

Exposure ulcers are therefore supposedly not a specific sequelae of the measles-keratitis, in contrast to the erosions.

It goes without saying that in some patients both factors – viral keratitis and exposure – can cooperate to cause corneal damage.

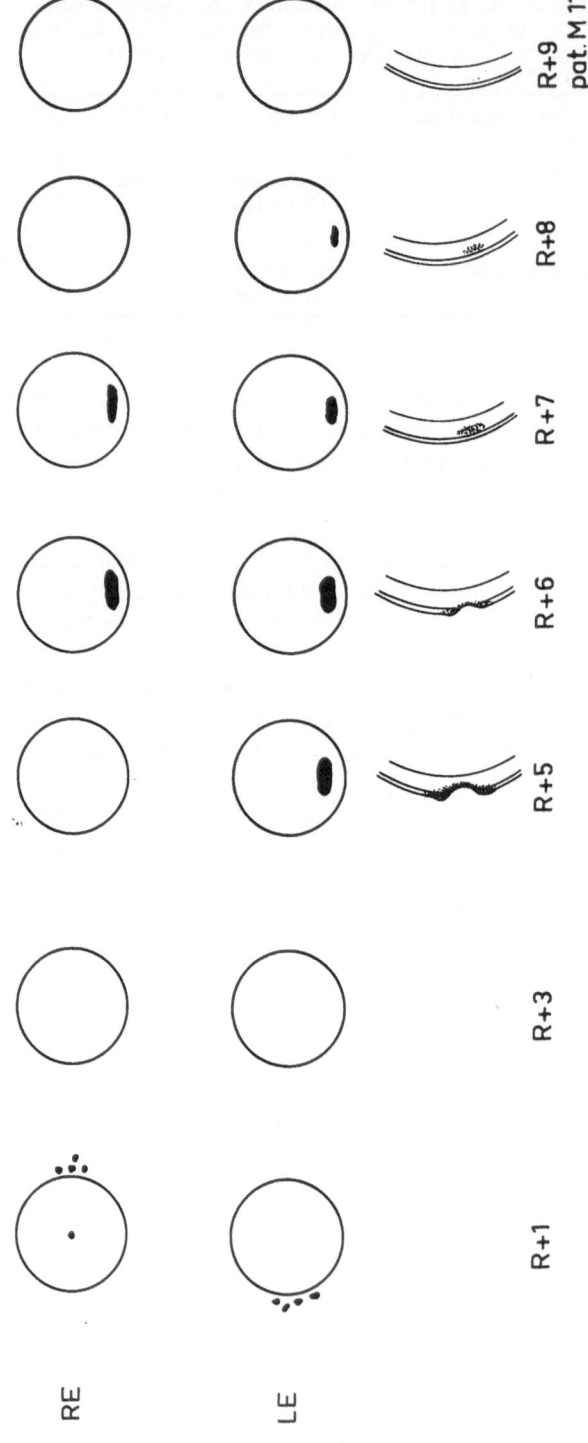

RE

LE

R+1   R+3   R+5   R+6   R+7   R+8   R+9
pat. M 117

Figure 4.2.2.b. The course of an exposure ulcer in a 5 year old boy with measles

4.3. The prophylactic value of tetracycline eye-ointment 1% and Vitamin A 200.000 iU

4.3.1. Measles-keratitis

In the first 148 patients we didn't interfere with the treatment as prescribed by the attending doctor. So 84 patients were prescribed tetracycline ointment because of the red aspect of their eyes.

At first sight it may seem confusing that the treated patients had a more severe keratitis than the non-treated children (average keratitis score 7 compared to 4). Probably this will only mean that the extent of the subepithelial conjunctivitis and the severity of the epithelial keratitis are associated.

In the clinical trial (Mukumu II and Kakamega) evaluation of tetracycline ointment as a prophylactic for the measles-keratitis was attempted. The numbers, however, were too small to allow for a statistical analysis. Anyhow, here no gross differences between the treated and non-treated eyes were observed.

It must also be said that it would be very unlikely that tetracycline ointment could have a preventive value against the viral measles-keratitis.

The limited numbers in our clinical trial also don't allow for any statement about the prophylactic value of Vitamin A, as far as the measles-keratitis is concerned.

4.3.2. Corneal erosions and exposure ulcers

In the whole group of 248 measles children 10 patients with corneal disease exceeding the common measles-keratitis were observed: 7 corneal erosions and 3 exposure ulcers. None of these corneal problems occurred in children who had received tetracycline eye-ointment. It is to be remembered that of the 148 children in Mukumu I, 84 children had received eye-ointment: generally they had a more severe keratitis, but did not develop corneal erosions. Since corneal erosions develop as an extension of the measles-keratitis, this is a surprising finding. In Mukumu II and Kakamega in every child one eye was protected with tetracycline eye-ointment. Both corneal erosions which were seen to develop during the observation-period occurred in unprotected eyes. The details of these 10 patients are given in fig. 4.3.2.

The same protective value of tetracycline eye-ointment 1% was observed in the safari-patients and no erosions or exposure ulcers were observed in children who had received eye-ointment. In many dispensaries the prescription of eye-ointment is a common routine measure for measles.

These observations demonstrate the prophylactic value of tetracycline eye-ointment in the prevention of erosions and exposure ulcers in early measles.

In table 4.3.2. one patient is to be found who developed a corneal erosion 3 days after the administration of 200,000 iU Vit A (fig. 4.2.1.a, see colour plate III).

46

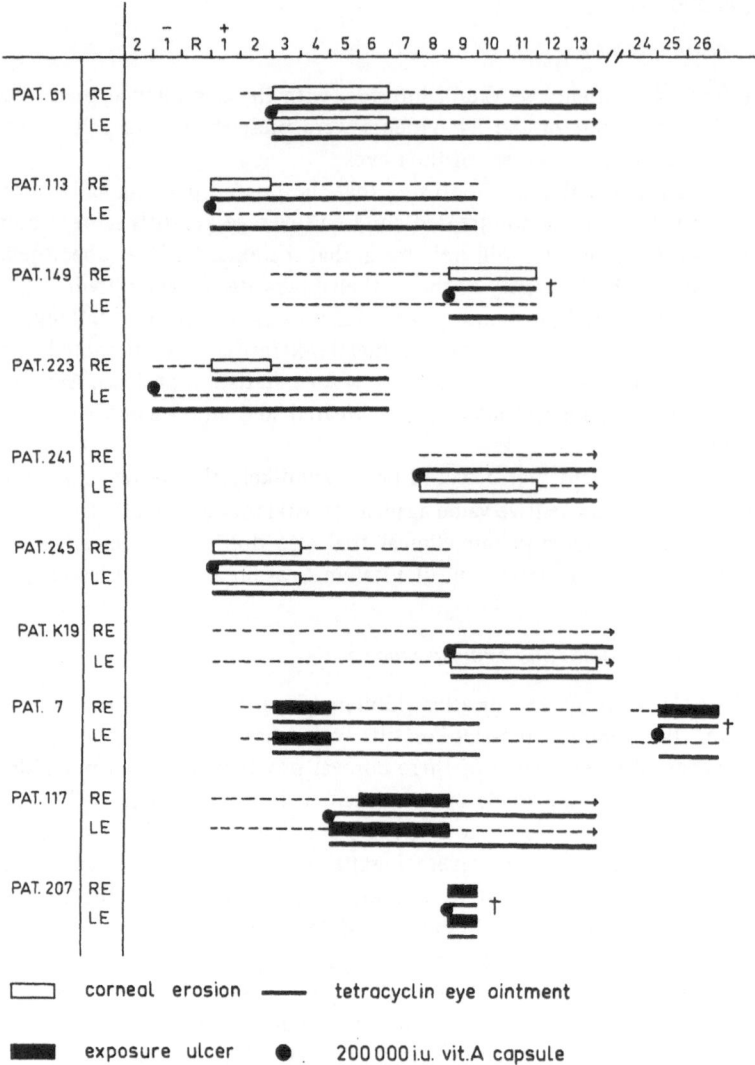

Figure 4.3.2. The occurrence of early corneal complications in children with measles in correlation with the time after outbreak of the rash (R) and the prescribed treatment. No erosions or exposure ulcers were seen to develop in eyes treated with tetracycline eye-ointment

This single observation does not allow a statement about the prophylactic value of Vitamin A in the prevention of corneal disease, because of the limited number of patients in the trial groups.

4.4. Late ocular complications

On our safaris and at the open Eye Clinic Mukumu, 9 patients were seen with late ocular complications after measles.

Late complications are defined as complications occurring after the acute stage of the measles, but within 3 months after the rash.

As always with work originating from the bush of developing countries, many interesting data are missing and follow-up examination is nearly always lacking. The available data regarding sex, age, time of outbreak of the rash and clinical appearance of the cornea are tabulated in table 4.4.a.

Pat Tamb VA 120. (fig. 4.4.b: see colour plate I).

This 6 year old boy was seen 2 weeks after the measles rash had come out. At the time of first examination he had a perforation at the 6 o'clock position in the cornea of the left eye. Traditional herbal medicines had been applied by his mother since one week. It was impossible to retrieve details about the treatment. The boy belonged by tribe to the Elgeyo's. According to Mulder

Table 4.4.a. Patients with late complications after measles.
Rash: the time after the outbreak of the rash in weeks (wk).
TM +: traditional herbal medicine was applied.
TB: Tuberculosis.
EM: Electron microscopy.

Number	Sex	Age in years	Rash	Clinical aspect of the cornea	Remarks
Tamb VA 120 (Fig. 4.4b)	M	6	2 wk	Perforation at 6 o'clock	TM +
Muk P 258 (Fig. 4.4c-d)	F	2.8/12	2 wk	RE: panophthalmitis LE: adhaerent leucoma	cornea EM TM + Fig. 5.3 d-h.
Tamb P 273 (Fig. 4.4e)	M	1.4/12	3 wk	Hypopyon ulcer	TM +
Chw P 172 (Fig. 3.3)	F	4	4 wk	Herpetic keratitis	TM +
Tamb VA 28 (Fig. 4.4f-g)	F	8	4 wk	RE: Perforated cornea LE: Phlyctaenular keratitis	TB
Muk VA 7	M	2.6/12	4 wk	Healing corneal ulcer	
Bus P 158	F	1.2/12	5 wk	Herpetic keratitis	
Sia VA 16 (Fig. 4.4h)	M	7/12	5 wk	Central corneal necrosis	
Bung VA 83 (Fig. 4.4i)	F	1.6/12	8 wk	Corneal staphyloma	

(personal communication) it is unthinkable that an Elgeyo mother will ever serve a meal to her family consisting of only "posho" (maize) without "mboga" (green leafy vegetable of any kind). This excludes more or less Vitamin A deficiency, of which also no other symptoms or signs were present.

It is remarkable that also the mother had an adhaerent leucoma in the left eye, which — according to her — had developed in connection with measles.

Pat Muk P 258. (fig. 4.4.c and d: see colour plate I).
This 2 year 8 month old, severely malnourished girl was seen at the open Eye Clinic Mukumu, 2 weeks after the rash. The right eye was lost because of a panophthalmitis. An evisceration was performed, a purulent hyalitis was found. The corneo-scleral rim was preserved for light and electron-microscopy. On electron-microscopical examination possibly measles virus was detected in the keratocytes (fig. 5.3.h). The left eye showed a descemetocele, with incarceration of iris.

Pat Tamb P 273. (fig. 4.4.e: see colour plate I).

This Elgeyo boy, 1 year and 4 months of age, was seen 3 weeks after the outbreak of the rash. The cornea of the right eye showed a small paracentral ulcer, and a secondary iritis with hypopyon was present. A smear was taken from the ulcer and Gram stained. No bacteria were seen in sufficient amounts to be blamed as the cause of the ulceration. The attending mother admitted the application of traditional medicines. It has been mentioned already that the application of herbs frequently gives rise to an iritis (Duke Elder and MacFaul, 1972). After treatment with atropine ointment, chloramphenicol ointment and pad and bandage, the ulcer healed and the hypopyon disappeared. 200.000 iU Vitamin A were also given.

Pat Chw P 172 (fig. 3.3: see colour plate I).
Luhya girl, 4 years of age. Herpetic keratitis, 4 weeks after the measles. Traditional medicines had been applied.

Pat Tamb VA 28. (fig. 4.4.f and g: see colour plate I).
This 8 year old Kalengin girl was seen for the first time 4 weeks after the rash. The girl made a lamentable impression; she was extremely photophobic and cried continuously. The scalp was covered with impetigo, bald areas alternated with the remaining red hair. The submandibular lymphnodes were swollen and tender. The chest X-ray was very suggestive for pulmonary tuberculosis. In the left eye several phlyctaenulae were visible; the cornea of the right eye had perforated at the six o'clock position. The child was treated with systemic antibiotics and tubercolustatics. The reaction to treatment was good. Four months later the child was seen again in consultation. The perforation in the right eye had healed with an adhaerent leucoma. The cornea of the left eye was clear.

Pat Sia VA 16. (fig. 4.4.h: see colour plate I).
This 7 month old boy was seen 5 weeks after the outbreak of the rash. The cornea of the left eye showed a central necrosis. The perforation was plugged off by the lens, the anterior chamber was virtually non-existent. The child

was lost for treatment and follow-up. No Bitot's spots were seen. The child was breastfed, supplemented with cow's milk.

Pat Bung VA 38. (fig. 4.4.i: see colour plate I).
This 18 month old girl was seen 2 months after the measles. The child was extremely well fed. The right eye showed a nearly total corneal staphyloma. No Bitot's spots were observed, and she did not complain about night blindness.

Pat Muk VA 7.
This $2\frac{1}{2}$ year old Luhya boy was seen with a corneal ulcer, 4 weeks after the measles rash. The ulcer had not perforated and was in transition to a corneal leucoma. No data regarding his nutritional status are available.

Pat P 158.
A 14 month old Luhya girl was seen with an herpetic keratitis, 5 weeks after the measles rash. No other data are available.

These late complications after measles are much more varied than the early ones. In some cases it was not possible to make a distinct etiological diagnosis, but supposedly the application of traditional medicines, tuberculosis and herpes are important etiological factors.

The nutritional data of these patients are given in table 6.4.

5 – Immunofluorescence-, light- and electron-microscopy of conjunctival biopsies and corneal specimens

In the previous paragraphs a clinical description was given of the subepithelial conjunctivitis and the epithelial conjunctivo-keratitis as signs of measles. This chapter will deal with the anatomical features of these conjunctival and corneal lesions.

Immunofluorescence for measles virus still gives positive results in skin biopsies up to 4 days after the outbreak of the rash, whereas measles virus can only be cultured exceptionally after 36–48 hours. Moreover, storage of specimens at 4°C for 48 hours does not influence the quality of the immunofluorescence tests in cryostate sections (Olding-Stenkvist and Bjorvatn, 1976). This means that immunofluorescence tests are less vulnerable than culturing techniques. A major advantage of immunofluorescence, important in view of the clinical differentiation made in the two conjunctival signs of measles, is the possibility to localize the virus.

Localization of virus by the electronmicroscope is a far more elaborate enterprise, but allows more detailed insight in the pathological processes occurring at the cellular level.

5.1. Immunofluorescence of conjunctival biopsies

5.1.1. Technique

After thawing, the specimens (§3.6) were taken out of the transport medium and snapfrozen in isopentane, chilled by liquid nitrogen. Cryostate sections of 1 μ thickness were cut on a Slee microtome.

The slides were coded and independently prepared and examined in two different laboratories: Dr. F.E. Nommensen of the Department of Virology and Dr. F.J.W. ten Kate of the Institute of Pathology, both at the Erasmus University, Rotterdam. Both laboratories used essentially the same techniques and materials.

The slides were air dried and stored at $-70°C$. The air dried specimens were fixed in acetone at $-20°C$ for 10 minutes. After air drying at room temperature the specimens were incubated for 45 minutes with commercially available F.I.T.C. (Fluorescein Iso Thiocyanate Conjugated) anti-measles-goat-serum (Microbiological Associates Inc. Walkersville, Maryland, USA) in an optimal 1:40 dilution. After washing in phosphate buffered saline, the slides were mounted in buffered glycerol 80% (pH 7.4) and examined under a Zeiss fluorescence microscope with incident ultraviolet light.

To assess the specificity of this technique, control experiments were done with the following results.

(a) Lissamine Green had no toxic effect on a Vero cell culture, (Green Monkey kidney cells) and did not influence the auto-fluorescence of these cells.

(b) Lissamine Green had no affinity to cells infected with a Schwarz measles strain in vitro:

(c) The undiluted conjugated serum did not stain respiratory syncytial virus, para-influenzavirus type 1, 2 and 3, mumps virus, influenza virus A and B, herpes simplex virus type I and adenovirus (not typed).

(d) Some slides were incubated with F.I.T.C. antiserum against adenovirus or herpes implex virus type I. Both experiments were negative.

These controls make it very likely that the fluorescence present in our slides demonstrates specifically the presence of measles virus antigen.

It was also tried to do immunofluorescence tests on Epon embedded material, after acid elution (Fulton and Middleton 1975), but all attempts failed to give positive results.

5.1.2. Results of the immunofluorescence tests on 5 conjunctival biopsies

The data regarding the children from whom the biopsies were taken are tabulated in table 5.1.2.a.

Culturing of the measles virus from these biopsies was tried, but all cultures stayed negative. This is not surprising in view of the time after the rash at which the biopsy was taken. In a single case (no. 3) a positive culture might have been possible, but probably here also the hazards of long-range-transportation and delay have influenced the negative outcome.

Together with the biopsies a venous bloodsample was drawn to assess the presence of anti-measles IgM. The technical difficulties appeared unsurmountable and no IgM estimations were performed on these sera.

Fig. 5.1.2.b (see colour plate III) demonstrates the presence of measles virus antigen in the subepithelial tissue.

In fig. 5.1.2.c (see colour plate III) an example of the immunofluorescence of the conjunctival epithelium is given. The fluorescent activity is localized in the cytoplasm and demonstrates specifically the presence of measles-virus-antigen.

Table 5.1.2.a. Sex, age of the children and time of biopsy taking in relation to the day of outbreak of the rash (R). These biopsies were sent to the Erasmus University Rotterdam for examination with immunofluorescent techniques.

Patient	Sex	Age in years	R
KNH 1	M	2	+ 3
KNH 2	M	6/12	+ 5
KNH 3	M	4	+ 1
KNH 4	F	1.1/12	+ 4
KNH 5	M	8/12	+ 4

Table 5.1.2.d. The distribution of antimeasles immunofluorescence in 5 paired conjunctival biopsies, staining and non-staining with Lissamine Green (LG + and LG −), performed by 2 different laboratories (Lab A = Dpt. of Virology; Lab B = Dpt. of Pathology, Erasmus University Rotterdam). In the Lissamine Green positive epithelial lesions measles antigene was present. In other biopsies viral activity was found subepithelially, as manifestation of the subepithelial conjunctivitis of prodromal measles.

		Epithelium		Subepithelium	
		Lab A	Lab B	Lab A	Lab B
Pat 1	LG +	+	+	−	−
	LG −	−	−	+	+
Pat 2	LG +	+	+	−	−
	LG −	−	−	+	?
Pat 3	LG +	+	+	−	−
	LG −	?	−	+	+
Pat 4	LG +	+	+	+	−
	LG −	−	−	−	+
Pat 5	LG +	+	+	−	−
	LG −	−	−	−	+

All results of the direct anti-measles immunofluorescence tests of both laboratories are tabulated in table 5.1.2.d.

From this table two conclusions are to be drawn.

(a) An excellent concordance exists between the results of both laboratories. It is to be remembered that these results were obtained on coded specimens, which makes the next conclusion even more reliable.

(b) In the specimens taken from Lissamine Green positive areas the measles virus is located in the epithelium; in the Lissamine Green negative areas no virus could be detected in the epithelium. In many of the LG negative areas viral activity was found in the subepithelial lymphoid tissue.

These findings fit into the previously described clincial distinction between a subepithelial conjunctivitis and an epithelial conjunctivo-keratitis.

It is of great importance that the viral nature of the conjunctivo-keratitis in measles could be proved by these observations and this may have far reaching consequences for our thinking about the pathogenesis of Post-Measles-Blindness.

5.2. Light- and electron-microscopy of conjunctival biopsies

5.2.1. Techniques

The 5 paired conjunctival biopsies and the corneal specimens (§3.6) were fixed in a mixture of glutaraldehyde and paraformaldehyde (Peters 1970).

For light-microscopy small pieces were embedded in paraplast; 7 μm

sections were stained with either periodic acid Schiff (PAS) or with hema-
toxylineosin (HE).

For electron-microscopy small blocks were postfixed for 1 hour in os-
miumtetroxyde (Palade 1955), dehydrated in graded series of ethanol and
subsequently embedded in Epon 812. Ultrathin sections were made on a
Reichert OmU 3 ultramicrotome, stained with uranylac:·tate and leadcitrate
and studied in a Philips EM 400.

In order to experience the normal appearance of measles virus under the
electronmicroscope, a measles infected Vero cell culture (Green Monkey
Kidney cells) served as a control. After centrifugation this cell culture was
treated in the same way as the conjunctival biopsies. Moreover, some thick
sections $(0.5\,\mu m)$ were investigated by a combined application of scanning
and transmission electronmicroscopy (STEM).

5.2.2. Light microscopy of conjunctival biopsies

The data regarding the patients from whom the biopsies were taken are
tabulated in table 5.2.2.a.

Epithelium

In many places the epithelium shows no abnormality: the cells are regularly
arranged, occasionally a goblet cell is seen between light and dark stained
apical cells. In many basal cells the cytoplasm contains melanosomes, arranged
at the apex of the nucleus.

In specimens, taken from Lissamine Green positive areas, the intercellular
spaces seem to be widened, and islands of epithelium are seen where cells are
desquamated (fig. 5.2.2.b., c and e); at some places hardly any epithelium
is left (fig. 5.2.2.d.)

These areas of desquamation showed a patchy distribution and were
bordered by areas of normal epithelium (fig. 5.2.2.e).

Some epithelial giant cells were observed.

In a single specimen, from a 1 year old girl (Bung P 265) with a conjunctival xerosis (but with no other signs and symptoms of Vitamin A deficiency), was also found a proliferation of the basal epithelium, with the

Table 5.2.2.a. Data regarding sex, age and day after outbreak of the
rash (R) at which conjunctival biopsies for pathology and eletron-
microscopy were taken from 5 measles patients.

Pat nr.	IOI nr.	Sex	R	Age in years	Remarks
M 223	77141	F	−2	1.9/12	
M 234	77143	F	+1	1	
Bung P 179	77142	F	+2	1.9/12	
Bung P 265	7841	F	+2	1	xerosis
Bus P 216	7839	M	+3	10/12	

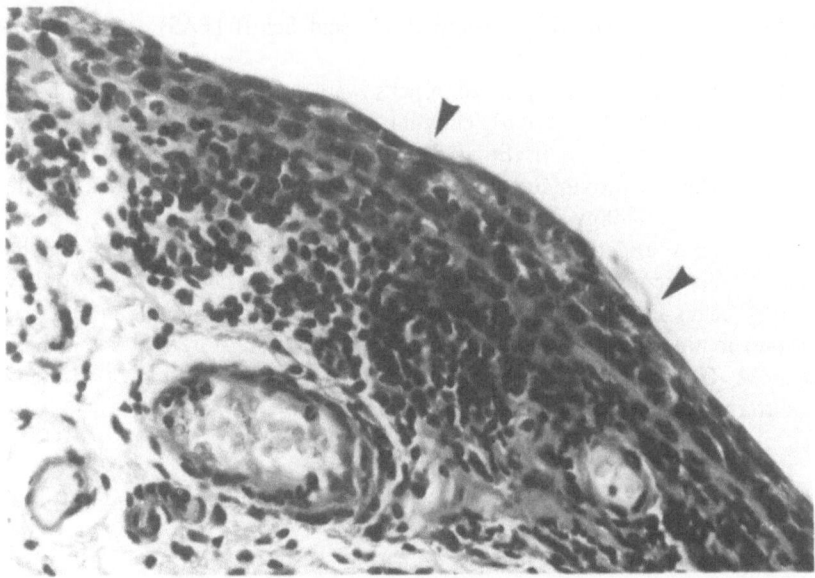

Figure 5.2.2.b. Conjunctiva: the central part of the epithelium (between arrowheads) shows loss of intercellular cohesion. Dyskeratotic and necrotic cells are seen. In the sub-epithelial tissue infiltration by mononuclear cells is present. Hematoxylin-Eosin × 100. Pat Bus P 216, Negative PA EUR 28092

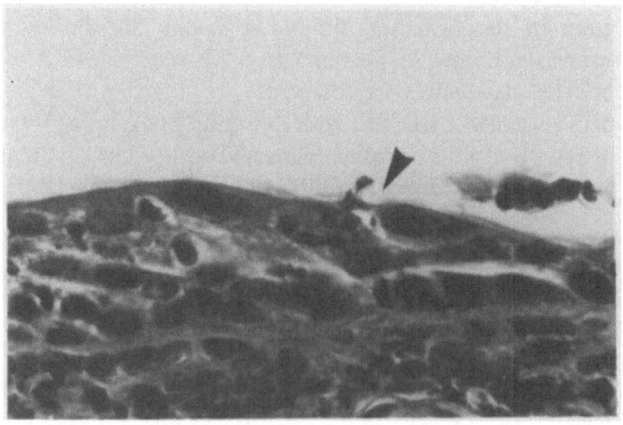

Figure 5.2.2.c. In the same patient, now at a higher magnification, the loss of inter-cellular adhesion is demonstrated by the presence of intercellular clefts (arrowhead). Hematoxylin-Eosin × 125. Negative PA EUR 28092

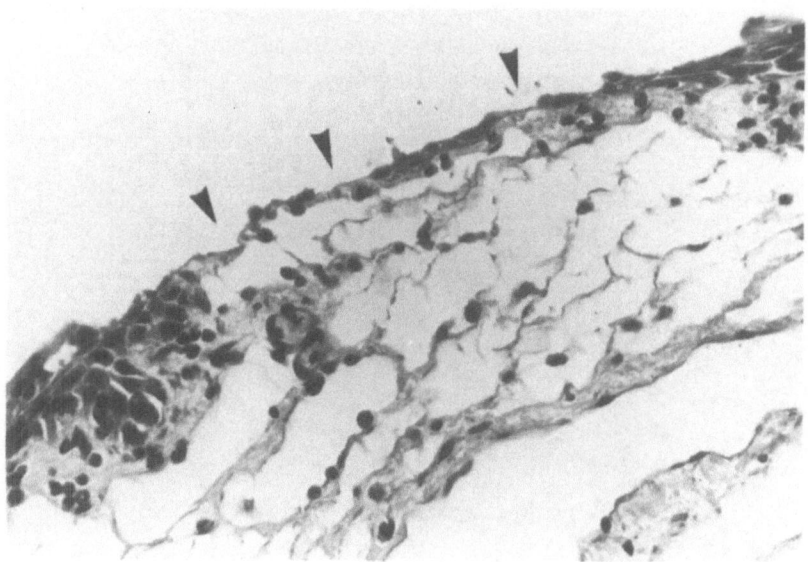

Figure 5.2.2.d. In this conjunctival biopsy (Pat Bung P 265) severe oedematous changes are present in the subepithelial tissue. In some places (arrowheads) all epithelium has vanished: the basement membrane is left bare. Hematoxylin-Eosin × 100, Negative PA EUR 28092

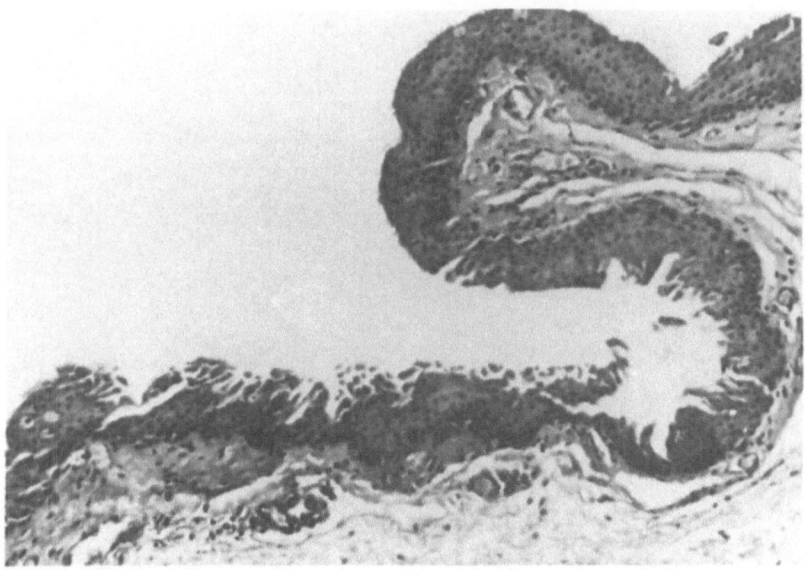

Figure 5.2.2.e. In this conjunctival biopsy the desquamation of the epithelium is seen to take place: on the left hand side the epithelium is desquamating, whereas on the right hand side the epithelium is normal. Hemtoxylin-Eosin × 40. Pat Bus P 216, Negative PA EUR 28092

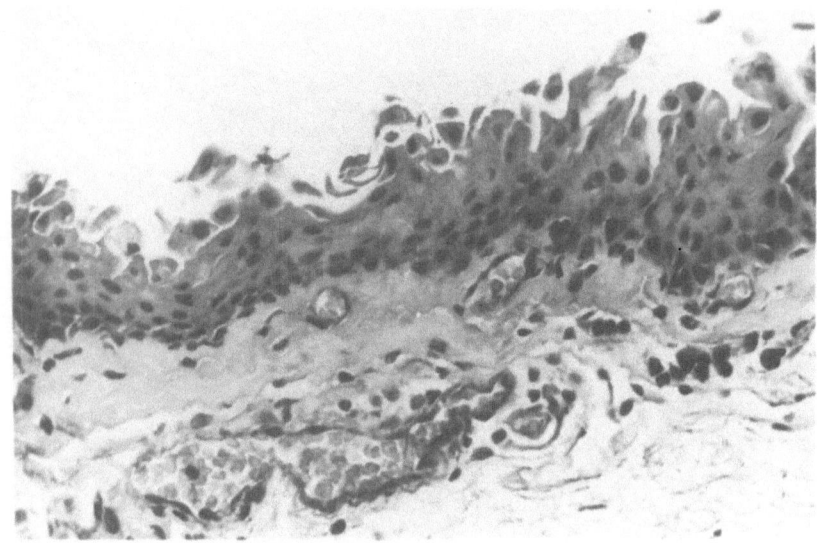

Figure 5.2.2.f. The same patient as the previous fig. The desquamating epithelium is seen at a higher magnification (× 100)

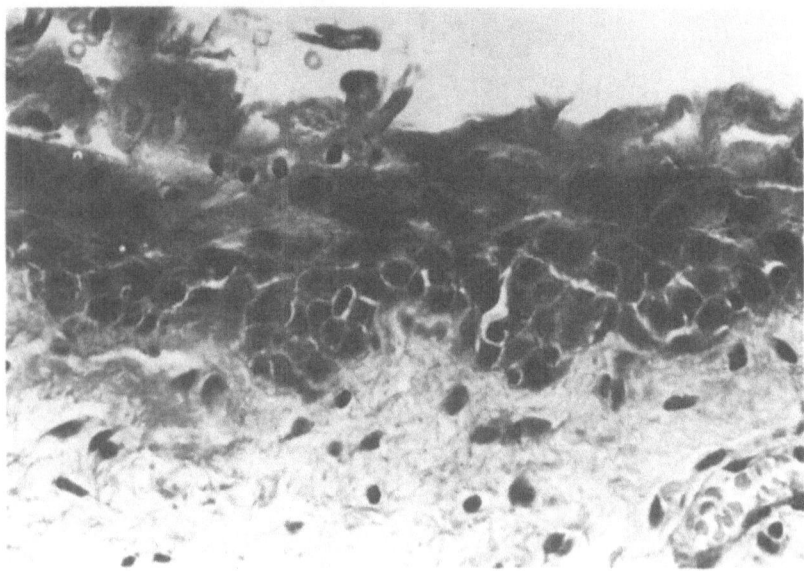

Figure 5.2.2.g. Conjunctival biopsy from a xerotic area: focal loss of coherence of epithelial cells with keratinization of superficial layers. The subepithelial tissue shows severe oedema. Pat Bung P 265, Hematoxylin-Eosin × 125. Negative PA EUR 28093

formation of pegs below the basement membrane. This was also the only specimen with signs of keratinization of the conjunctival epithelium (fig. 5.2.2.g).

Inclusion bodies were not observed in any of the specimens.

Substantia propria

In most cases the substantia propria underlying the epithelium showed little signs of inflammation. In other biopsies a severe oedema (fig. 5.2.2.d) is present. A moderate vasodilation is seen in other specimens. Occasionally an infiltration by mononuclear cells is observed. No inclusion bodies or giant cells were found.

5.2.3. Electron microscopy of conjunctival biopsies

Epithelium

Many areas with normal epithelium are observed. The epithelial cells show the characteristic ultrastructural features, the microvilli extend from the apical cell membrane, the nuclear chromatin is condensed at the nuclear border.

In other places degenerating cells with pycnotic nuclei are found. The cytoplasm of the apical cells seems relatively empty: inside the cytoplasm mitochondria, ribosomes and endoplasmic reticulum are unevenly distributed. A prominent feature is the presence of dilated intercellular spaces. The lateral cell membrane shows its typical deep indentations, studded with desmosomes, which seem to link the cells together, even when the intercellular spaces are strongly dilated (fig. 5.2.3.a). Occasionally a goblet cell is seen (fig. 5.2.3.b).

Substantia propria

The collagen fibrils are irregularly oriented and in some cases clumped together to form amorphous structures. In between this collagen many cells are observed, mainly plasma cells, lymphocytes and macrophages; occasionally polymorphonuclear leucocytes are seen (fig. 5.2.3.c). The cytoplasm contains an often swollen endoplasmic reticulum. Multivesicular bodies and bristle coated vesicles (which resemble lysosomal structures) are seen in great numbers.

In the cytoplasm cytoplasmic aggregates and accumulations of filamentous material are present (fig. 5.2.3.d). These strands measured 20 nm in thickness and resemble the strands found in measles infected vero cells (fig. 5.2.3.e and f)(cfr fig. 2.2.b). This finding suggests that the granular material inside the cells is of a viral nature.

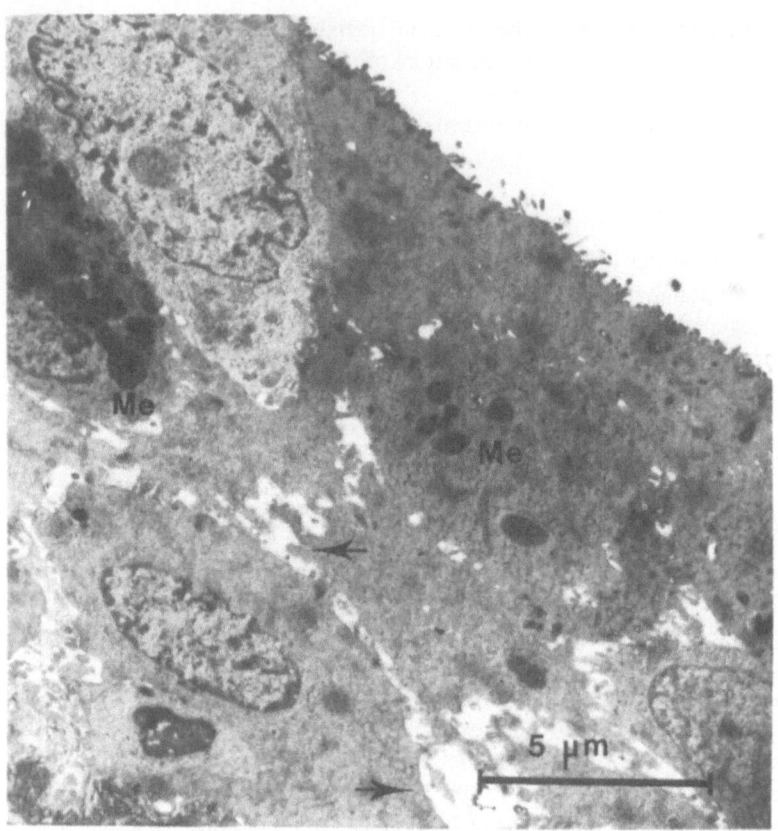

Figure 5.2.3.a. Electronmicroscopy of conjunctival epithelium. The apical cell border of the superficial cells shows characteristic microvilli. The cytoplasm of the cells differs markedly in electron density, melanin granules (Me) are frequently observed. The intercellular spaces are dilated (arrow). Pat M 234, Negative IOI 79088, magnification 6900 ×

Figure 5.2.3.b. Electron micrograph of a goblet cell (G) between epithelial cells with the adjacent part of the stroma. In the cytoplasm, numerous spherical globules with different electron densities are seen. Pat M 234, Negative IOI 79058, Magnification 6900 ×

Figure 5.2.3.c. Electron micrograph of a polymorphonuclear leucocyte in the conjunctival stroma. The cytoplasm contains numerous vesicles of lysosomal nature: large autophagic vacuoles (AV) and electron-dense bodies (EDB). The nuclear lobes (NUC) are indicated with arrowheads. Pat Bung P 265, negative IOI 79117, magnification 5900 ×

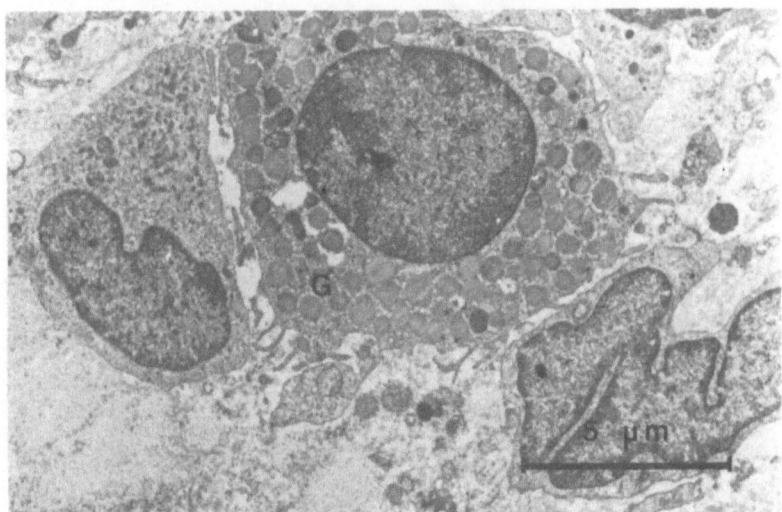

Figure 5.2.3.b.

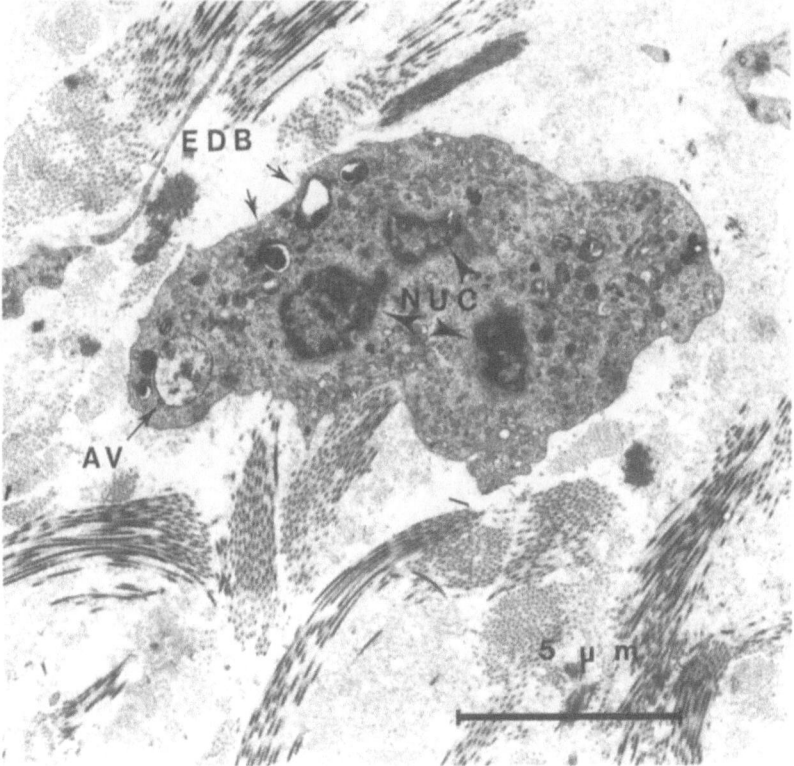

Figure 5.2.3.c.

60

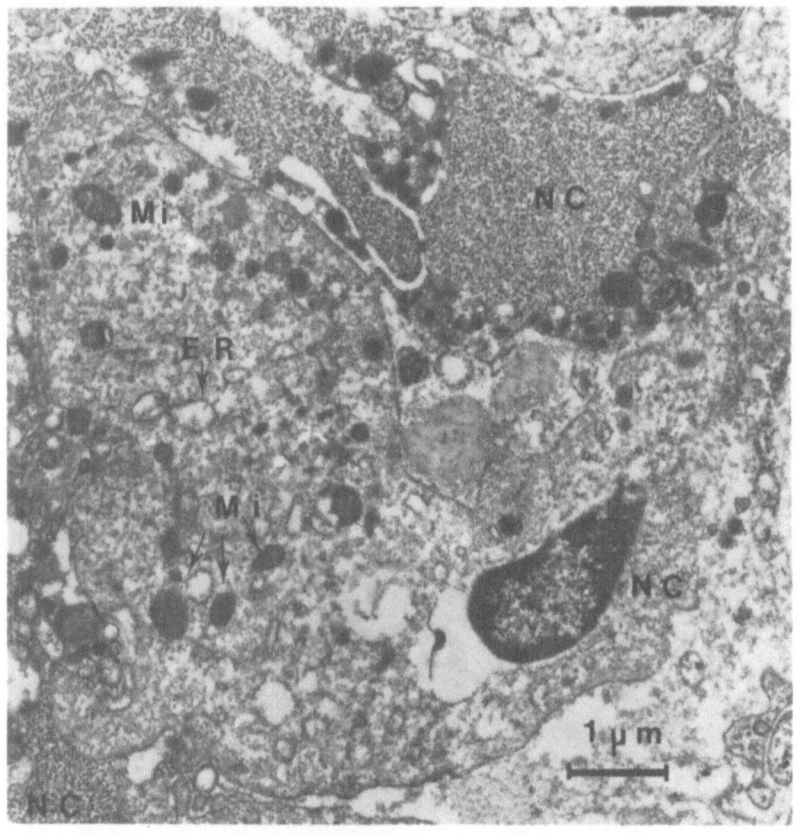

Figure 5.2.3.d. Electron micrograph at high magnification of a lymphocyte in the conjunctival stroma. Dark mitochondria (Mi) and a swollen endoplasmic reticulum (ER) are seen in the cytoplasm. Note the fine filamentous material, which may be viral nucleocapsid (NC). Pat M 234, Negative IOI 79023, magnification 15040 ×

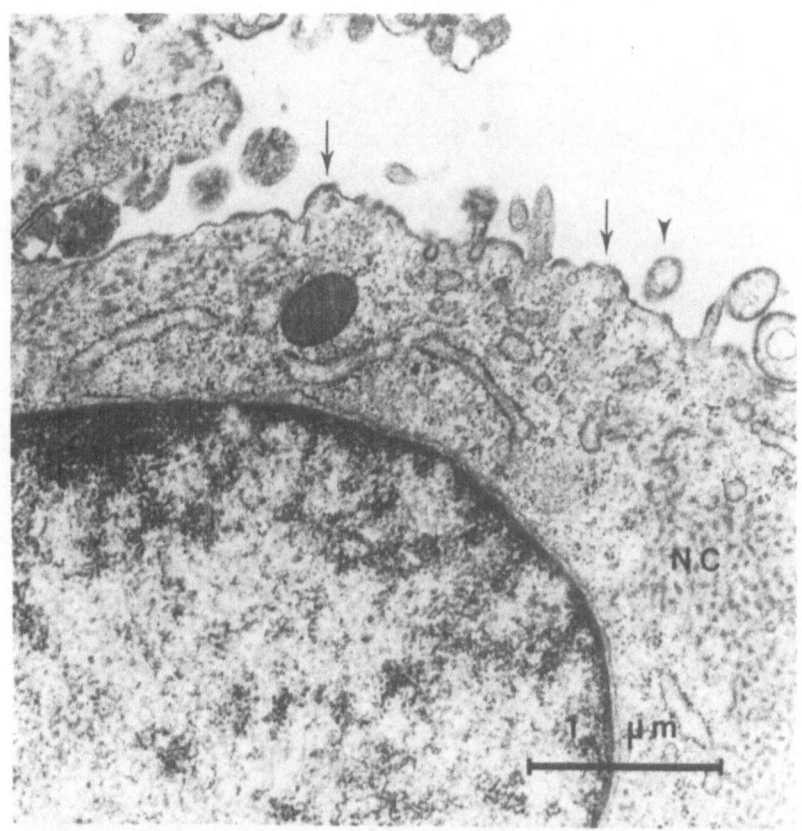

Figure 5.2.3.e. Scanning transmission electron micrograph of a cultured vero cell, infected with measles vaccine. The nucleocapsid (NC) is clearly visible. A virion (arrowhead) is seen with the fuzzy coat. The cellular membrane shows in several places a slight increase in cell coat (arrows) material. Negative IOI 79304, magnification 28600 ×

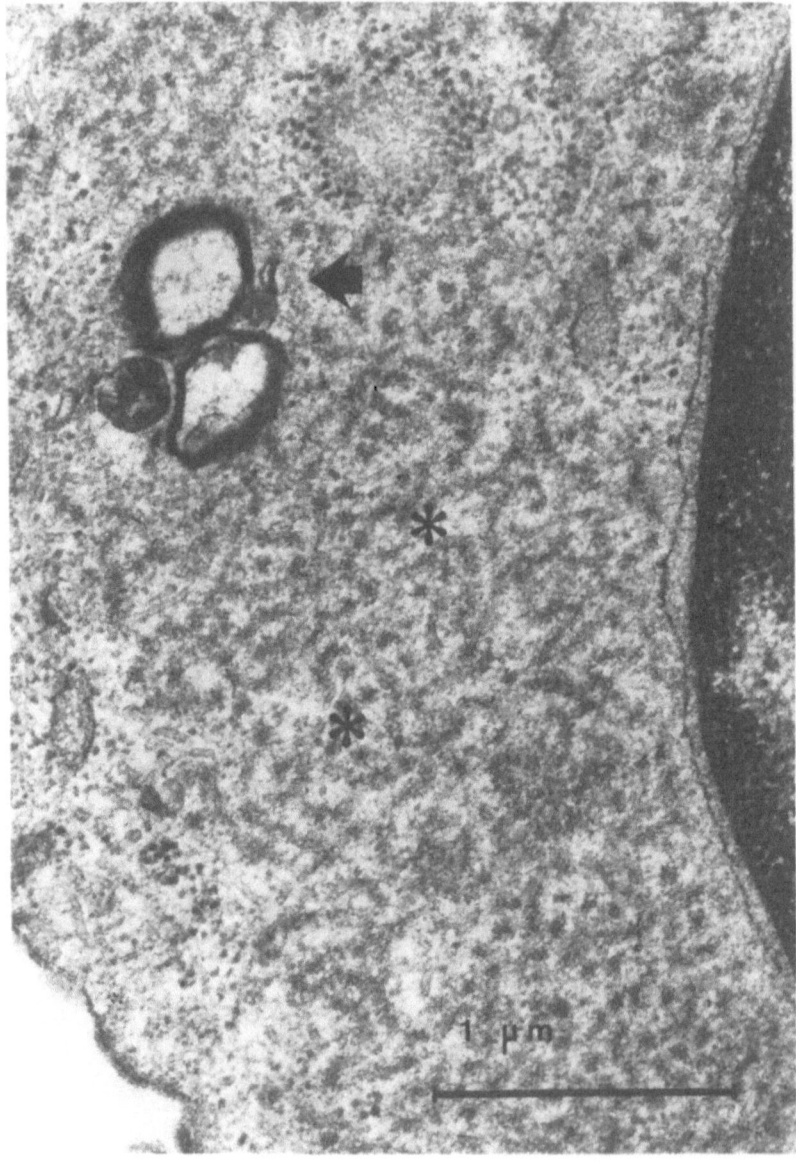

Figure 5.2.3.f. Scanning transmission electron micrograph shows part of a cultured cell after infection with measles vaccine. The cytoplasmis densely packed with nucleocapsid-aggegrates (asterix) and some degenerated membranous structures (arrow) are found. Negative IOI 790496, magnification 50400 ×

5.3. Light and electron microscopy of corneal specimens

Three corneal specimens were available for study under the microscope. The data regarding the patients are given in table 5.3.a.

Epithelium

In all 3 specimens the corneal epithelium showed essentially the same features as found in the conjunctival epithelium. At some places the epithelial cells show microvilli at the apical surface, covered by a fine thin filamentous layer, whereas in other parts the epithelium has diminished in thickness, and at some places even only some cell fragments on Bowman's membrane are left (fig. 5.3.b. and c). The intercellular spaces are again widely dilated. The anterior part of the epithelium only shows few cytoplasmic organelles: mitochondria, rough endoplasmic reticulum and Golgi apparatus are scarcely found.

Stroma

No abnormalities were observed in Bowman's membrane. In most cases the corneal collagen is normally arranged in bundles with uninterrupted periodicity. No signs of collagen breakdown were found.

Marked changes were found in the cornea with the perforation. Fig. 5.3.d gives the light microscopy. The scar of the corneal perforation is visible, with incarcerated iris pigment. An electronmicroscopical specimen taken from the newly formed scar-collagen, demonstrates the irregular arrangement of the collagen fibres. (fig 5.3.e.)

In the area of the microscopically unaltered cornea the collagen bundles have retained their normal periodicity. Here however many abnormal keratocytes are found. The cytoplasm of these cells contains swollen mitochondria and large vacuoles and fat inclusion bodies. Celllysis is frequently present, together with disruption of cytoplasmic membranes. Occasionally fine filamentous material, which shows great similarities to the viral strands in the cultured vero cells, can be seen. (fig 5.3.f, g and h)

Table 5.3.a. Data regarding sex, age and time after the outbreak of the rash (R) of the patients with corneal complications after measles, whose corneae were available for pathological examination.

Patient	IOI	Sex	Age in years	R	Corneal condition	Figure
M 149	7702	M	1.6/12	+ 11	Central macro-erosion	4.2.1.b-c,
M 207	77139	M	2.6/12	+ 10	Exposure ulcer	
Muk P258	7838	F	2.8/12	+ 14	Corneal perforation	4.4.c and d.

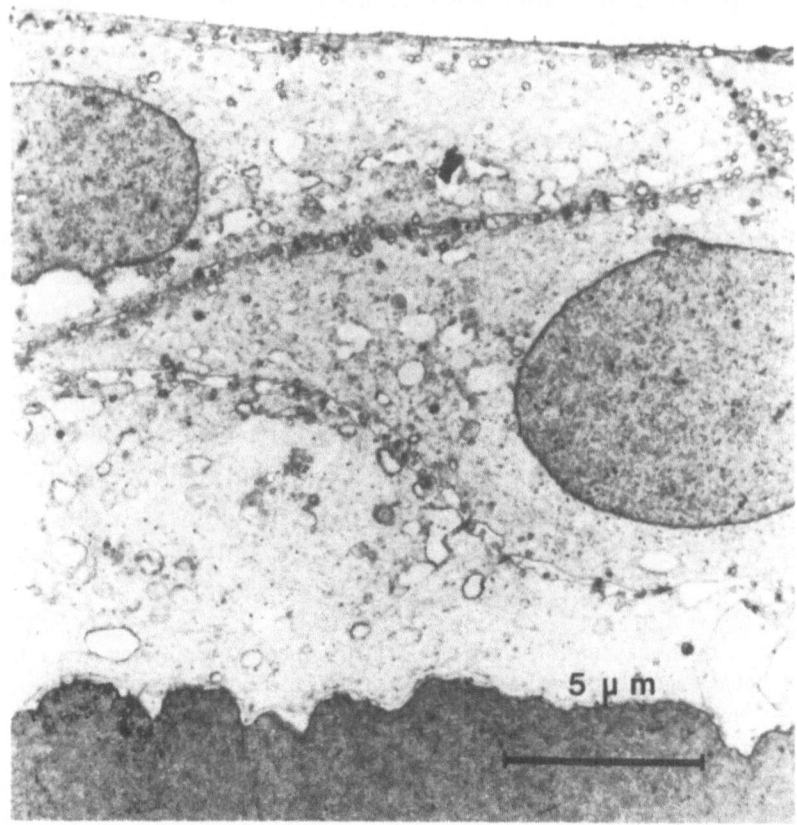

Figure 5.3.b. Electron micrograph of the corneal epithelium. The number of epithelial cell-layers is reduced. The apical cell surface is lacking microvilli, numerous cytoplasmic vecuoles can be observed. The basal lamina is intact. Pat M 149, Negative IOI 78418, magnification 6160 ×

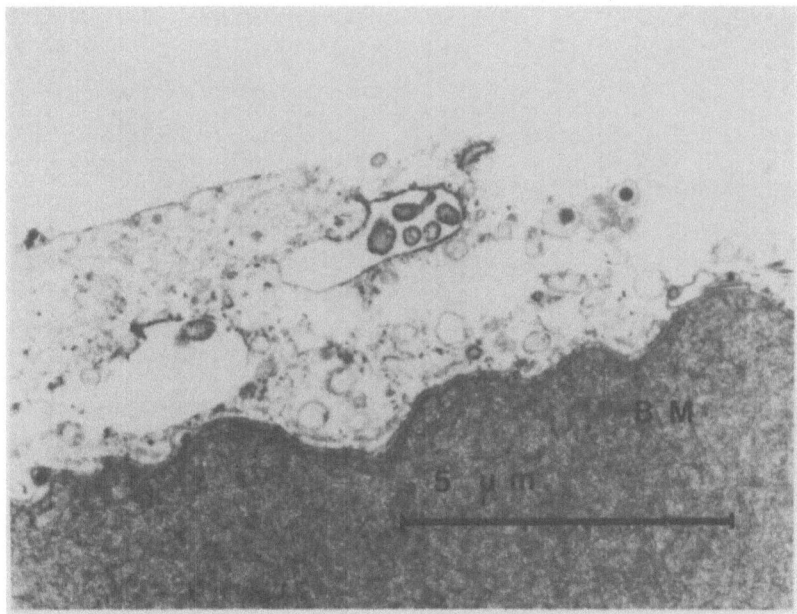

Figure 5.3.c. Electron micrograph of the corneal epithelium of a patient with a corneal erosion: most of the epithelial cells have disappeared, only some disrupted membranes are found. Bowman's membrane (BM) is lightly wrinkled. Pat M 149, Negative IOI, magnification 10,560 ×

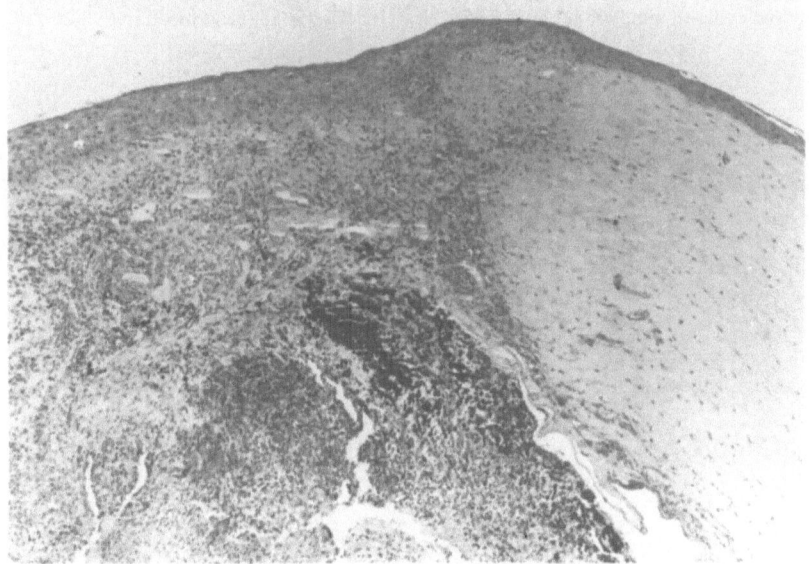

Figure 5.3.d. Scar of corneal perforation with incarcerated iris pigment epithelium. This patient was seen 2 weeks after the outbreak of the measles rash. The $2\frac{1}{2}$ year old girl was severely malnourished. The clinical impression "panophthalmitis" was confirmed on operation (fig. 4.4.c and d). Pat Muk P 258, Hematoxylin-Eosin × 16, Neg PA EUR 28093

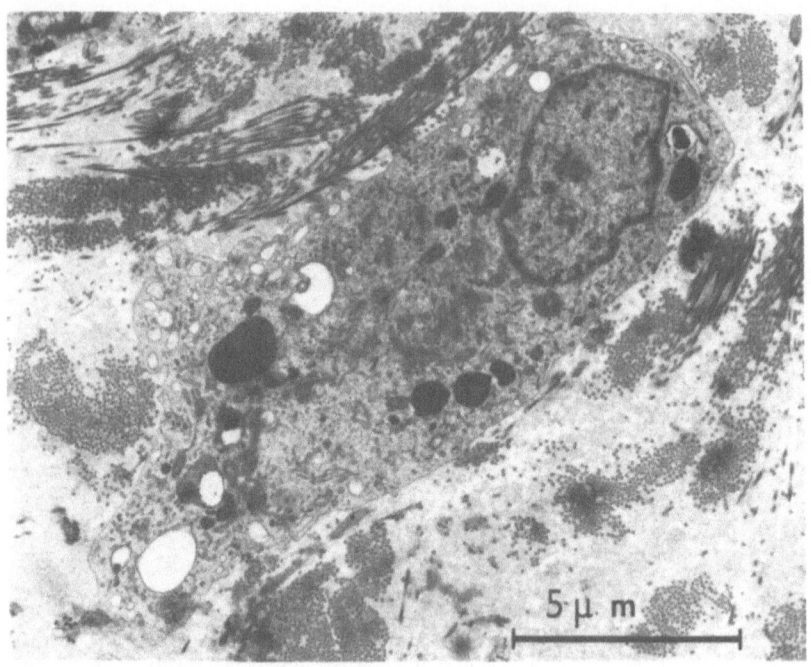

Figure 5.3.e. Electron micrograph of the scar of the perforation. A lymphocyte with numerous cytoplasmic electron dense vesicles is found in between the irregularly arranged collagen bundles. Pat Muk P 258, Negative IOI 79088, magnification 6900 ×

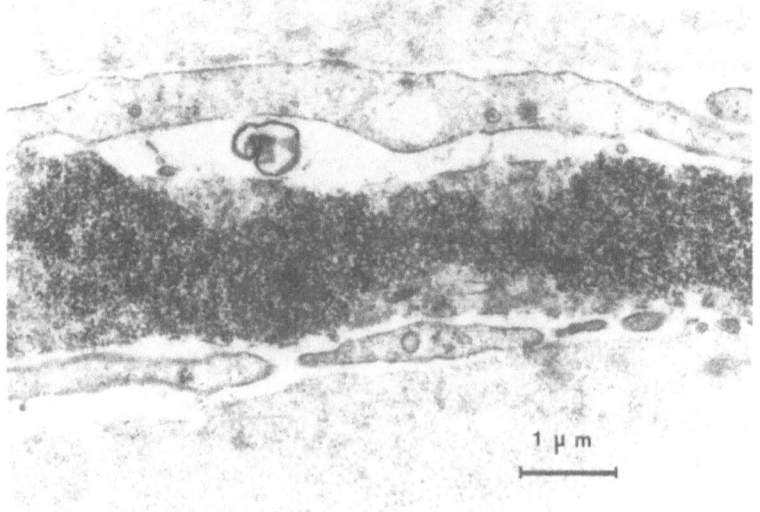

Figure 5.3.g. The same electron dense material as seen in the previous figure, now at a higher magnification. Pat Muk P 258, Negative IOI 8000257, magnification 22,000 ×

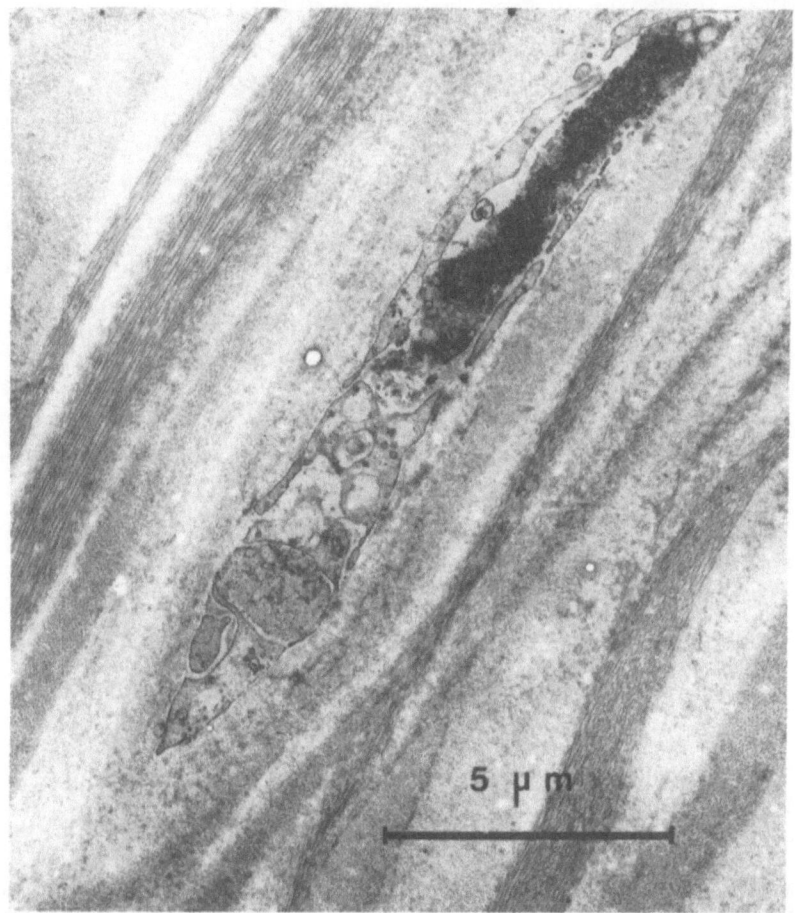

Figure 5.3.f. Electron micrograph of the normal corneal stroma of the perforated eye. The collagen bundles are regularly oriented. A large keratocyte is observed. In between the pseudopode-like protrusions of the keratocyte fine electron dense material is seen. Pat Muk P 258, Negative IOI 800256, magnification 78 0 ×

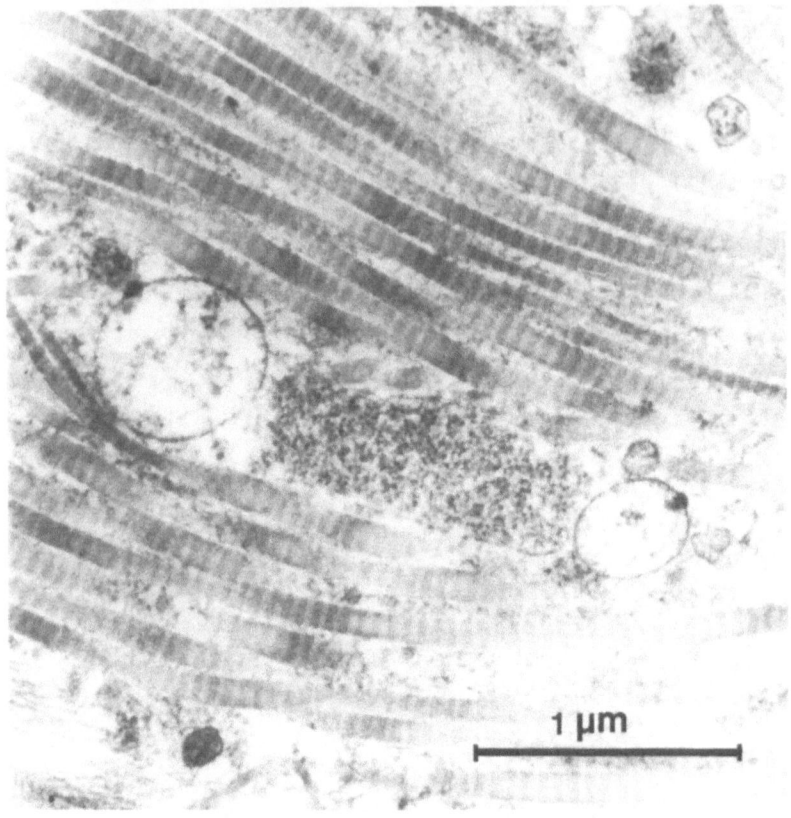

Figure 5.3.h. Electron micrograph at high magnification of the corneal stroma of the perforated eye. The collagen bundles show the normal periodicity. Note the fine filamentous material in between these bundles, resembling viral material (cfr fig. 5.2.3.e and g). Pat Muk P 258, Negative IOI 79017, magnification 64000   X

5.4. Discussion

The immunofluorescence tests on the conjunctival epithelium demonstrated the presence of measles antigen. Also the patchy distribution of these lesions is in concordance with the clinical findings. This leads to the conclusion that in the clinically observed epithelial lesions the measles virus plays a prominent role. No explanation can be given for the preferential localization of these lesions in the exposed parts of the bulbar conjunctiva.

No giant cells or inclusion bodies were observed. It is to be realized, however, that inclusion bodies and giant cells need some days to develop (Czajkowsky and Heneen 1976). Probably the time between the first appearance of these lesions and the taking of the biopsy was just too short for such a development. For the same reason it need not be surprising that in the electronmicroscope no viral strands were found, whereas viral antigen was observed in the cytoplasm by immunofluorescence. Immunofluorescence is a far more sensitive technique than light or electronmicroscopy. Further information could well be given by the use of ferritin labeled antiserum on specimens for electronmicroscopy.

The involvement of the conjunctival stroma in the measles infection is — at the time when biopsies were taken — of a much longer duration. This gives the time to develop the morphological correlates of the viral activity: viral strands were seen in the electronmicroscope, together with positive immunofluorescence.

Here also, no giant cells were found. It might be possible that the significance of measles giant cells in "normal" measles is exaggerated. Also Olding-Stenkvist and Bjorvatn (1976) reported a low incidence (cfr Roberts and Bain 1958).

In conclusion: the findings of the immunofluorescence and light- and electronmicroscopy fully support the distinction clinically made between the two conjunctival signs of measles: an early prodromal subepethelial conjunctivitis and an epithelial conjunctivo-keratitis occurring at the time of the rash.

One conjunctival biopsy was (on purpose) taken from a (non-staining) xerotic area. In the light microscopy keratinization of the superficial epithelium and the development of a rete peg were observed. Both changes are considered specific for a Vitamin A deficiency, as found in an experimental animal study by Pfister and Renner (1978).

These changes occurred only in this one specimen, selected on clinical grounds, as with a conjunctival xerosis measles-patient. The microscopy is totally different from the one seen in measles: measles conjunctivitis and Vitamin A deficiency are two, totally different, entities.

The conjunctival and corneal epithelium showed the same pathological changes: a diminished epithelial adhesiveness leading to patchy desquamation of the epithelium. In my opinion this is also to be considered as the cause of the high incidence of corneal erosions in measles-keratitis (cfr Khodadoust et al. 1968; Fogle et al. 1975).

Inside the keratocytes of the perforated cornea a granular material was found. It shares some morphological characteristics with viral RNA strands, and it is very attractive to suppose that this material indeed represents measles virus. In my opinion it is not allowed to state this positively. A study of the cornea with ferritin-labeled antiserum is badly needed

70

6 – The nutritional status of the children with measles-keratitis and corneal complications

In the literature not only complications of measles are consistently associated with malnutrition, but also the signs of measles are more severe in malnourished children (§2.5).

For this study the same might apply and the question arises whether the ocular signs of measles (i.e. the measles-keratitis) are more severe in children in a worse nutritional state. A positive association would be very significant in view of the fact that blinding complications of measles occur more frequently in malnourished children.

In order to test the hypothesis of a possible association between the measles-keratitis and nutritional status a quantitative classification for the keratitis was devised (§3.3). This classification was compared with age, sex, history of immunization and anthropometric and biochemical parameters of the nutritional status. In the next paragraphs the tables will be given. In all tables the χ^2-test was used for the statistical analyses.

6.1. Measles-keratitis and age, sex and history of immunization

In table 6.1.a the age of 126 measles patients and the classification for measles-keratitis are compared. No association exists.

In table 6.1.b the sex of the measles children and their keratitis classification are compared. Again, no statistical association was detected. In table 6.1.c the immunization history against measles is compared with the measles-keratitis. These two data are not associated. It is to be remembered however that the data regarding vaccination have only very limited value: the memory of the mother may be at fault (measles vaccination doesn't leave a specific scar like cowpox and BCG) and the vaccination itself may be of a bad quality:

Table 6.1.a. The age of 126 measles patients and the classification for measles-keratitis. No association existed between the age of the measles children and the extent of the measles-keratitis

| Age in months | Keratitis classification | | | | | |
	I	II	III	IV	V	Total
0–12	5	5	6	6	4	26
13–24	7	12	6	6	10	41
25–36	7	7	6	4	5	29
37 +	6	6	5	6	7	30
total	25	30	23	22	26	126

$\chi^2_{12} = 4.01 \quad p = 0.98$

71

Table 6.1.b. The sex and the classification for measles-keratitis in 124 measles patients. No association was observed between the sex of measles children and the extent of the measles-keratitis

Sex	Keratitis classification					Total
	I	II	III	IV	V	
Male	12	15	9	13	10	59
Female	13	15	13	9	15	65
total	25	30	22	22	25	124

$x_4^2 = 2.21$ $p = 0.70$

Table 6.1.c. The history of vaccination against measles and the classification for measles-keratitis in 103 measles patients. No statistically significant association existed between the history of vaccination and the keratitis

Vaccination against measles	Keratitis classification					Total
	I	II	III	IV	V	
+	3	5	1	5	2	16
−	16	18	18	13	22	87
total	19	23	19	18	24	103

$x_4^2 = 5.21$ $0.20 < p < 0.30$

in developing countries it is very difficult to maintain the "cold chain" necessary for the transport of the vaccine to keep its effectivity.

Anyhow, no association was found between the measles-keratitis and sex, age and immunization history. These factors therefore don't have to be taken into account in the following statistical analysis of possible association of the measles-keratitis and nutritional status.

6.2. Measles-keratitis and nutritional status

To assess the nutritional status of our measles children anthropometric and biochemical parameters were used (§3.5). In table 6.2.a the Weight for Age, in table 6.2.b the Height for Age, in table 6.2.c the Weight for Height is compared with the keratitis classification. No statistical association was found between the measles-keratitis and these anthropometric parameters of nutritional status.

The same applies to the biochemical parameters of malnutrition: Serum Albumin and Retinol Binding Protein. The numbers are given in table 6.2.d and 6.2.e.

In conclusion: no statistical association could be detected between the extent and severity of the early virus related features of measles-keratitis and nutritional status in this group of 148 children.

Table 6.2.a. The Weight for Age of 105 measles patients and the classification for measles-keratitis. No association was observed

Weight for Age	Keratitis classification					Total
	I	II	III	IV	V	
≤ 60%	1	2	1	1	0	5
61–80%	8	7	13	12	12	52
≥ 81%	11	13	8	4	12	48
total	20	22	22	17	24	105

$$x_8^2 = 9.33 \quad 0.30 < p < 0.50$$

Table 6.2.b. The Height for Age of the measles patients and the measles-keratis. The extent of measles-keratitis was independent of the nutritional status – measured as Height for Age – of the measles children

Height for Age	Keratitis classification					Total
	I	II	III	IV	V	
≤ 90%	7	11	4	5	8	35
≥ 91%	13	12	17	10	16	68
total	20	23	21	15	24	103

$$x_4^2 = 4.07 \quad 0.30 < p < 0.50$$

Table 6.2.c. The Weight for Height of the measles patients and the measles-keratitis. No association exists between the weight for height of the measles children and the extent of the measles-keratitis

Weight for Height	Keratitis classification					Total
	I	II	III	IV	V	
≤ 90	7	8	9	6	13	43
91–100	4	4	5	8	2	23
≥ 101	7	10	6	2	9	34
total	18	22	20	16	24	100

$$x_8^2 = 12.03 \quad 0.10 < p < 0.20$$

6.3. The nutritional status of 10 children with early corneal complications

10 out of the 248 measles patients developed more severe corneal disease: 7 corneal erosions, 3 exposure ulcers. The data regarding the nutritional status of these patients are tabulated in table 6.3. For reasons of comparison, of all parameters the median values in our sample are given.

A statistical analysis of this table is self-evidently not possible, because of the limited number of patients.

Table 6.2.d. The classification for measles-keratitis and the serum albumin content in 100 measles patients. (normal value: 3,500–5,500 mg%.) No association is observed.

Serum albumin in mg%	Keratitis classification					Total
	I	II	III	IV	V	
≤ 2,500	7	6	6	3	5	27
2,501–3,000	5	5	10	7	5	32
≥ 3,000	8	11	4	9	9	41
total	20	22	20	19	19	100

$x_8^2 = 7.65 \quad 0.30 < p < 0.50$

Table 6.2.e. The measles-keratitis and the content of Retinol Binding Protein in the serum of 103 measles patients. (normal value: 3–6 mg%.). No association was found between the serum RBP and the extent of the measles keratitis.

RBP in serum in mg%	Keratitis classification					Total
	I	II	III	IV	V	
≤ 1.2	6	5	5	5	9	30
1.3–2.2	10	11	13	9	8	51
≥ 2.3	4	6	3	6	3	22
total	20	22	21	20	20	103

$x_9^2 = 5.41 \quad 0.70 < p < 0.80$

Table 6.3. Anthropometric and biochemical parameters for the nutritional status of 10 patients with corneal erosions and exposure ulcers. For comparative reasons the median values of the patients Mukumu I are given. The age is given in years; W/A = Weight for Age; H/A = Height for Age; W/H = Weight for Height; RBP = Retinol Binding Protein, normal value: 3–6 mgr%; Alb = Serum Albumin, normal value: 3,500–5,500 mgr%

Pat	Age	W/A	H/A	W/H	RBP	Alb
Central corneal erosions						
M 61	1 2/12	93	92	109	< 1.2	1995
M 113	3	78	91	91	1.3	2715
M 149[†]	1 6/12	80	92	90	2.4	3390
					1.2	3015
M 223	1 9/12	70	91	80	nd	nd
M 241	7/12	83	83	139	2.5	2425
M 245	9/12	80	99	83	nd	nd
K 19	2 2/12	71	87	87	2.7	3128
Exposure ulcers						
M 7[†]	4	63	93	72	1.2	< 1500
M 117	5 6/12	78	91	98	1.7	2790
						2595
M 207[†]	2 6/12	malnutrition			< 1.2	1850
Median value						
	1 9/12	80	93	95	1.5	2680

This table 6.3 however contains some noteworthy details.

(a) The children with corneal erosions seem to be the younger ones. This would be remarkable since the erosions are to be considered as effects of keratitis, but the keratitis itself is independent of the age.

(b) Exposure ulcers occur preferably in children in a bad condition and are accompanied by a high mortality. This finding is not unexpected and confirms the clinical impression.

(c) Of patient M 149 two serum samples were taken: the first on admission at day $R + 3$, the second at day $R + 9$ when the corneal erosion developed.

In both samples serum albumin was normal, albeit lower in the second one. The serum RBP had however dropped dramatically. This confirms again the value of fast reacting transport proteins as indicators of the nutritional status, not in a static anthropometric sense, but as a dynamic situation.

This is therefore a good example of the nutritional "disadaptation" in the wake of measles. Also, in both samples the IgM was negative, possibly again an example of a disturbed protein synthesis.

6.4. Nutritional status of patients with late corneal complications

In this study 9 patients with late corneal complications were seen. This number was low, because of the strict criteria used for inclusion into this study. Also a presumably higher mortality in children with corneal complications has to be taken into account.

The data regarding tribe, corneal appearance and the nutritional status (as far as available) are tabulated in table 6.4. Self-evidently, no statistical analysis of these data will be possible.

It is however remarkable, that only a limited number of data are indicative for malnutrition.

6.5. Discussion

Measles-keratitis

The lack of association between measles-keratitis and nutritional status is a rather surprising finding. The connection between malnutrition and impaired defense mechanisms might easily result in a higher virusload and therefore give rise to a more severe (because viral) keratitis.

A false negative result however is not to be excluded. Two possibilities exist to explain such a false negative result.

a. Underrepresentation of malnutrition

It has been described already (§3.7) that our patients form a representative

Table 6.4. (extension of table 4.4.a) Data regarding the sex, age and tribe of 9 patients with late corneal complications after measles

Sex	Age in years	Tribe	Corneal appearance	TM	Nutritional status	Fig.	Remarks
M	6	Elgeyo	Descemetocele	+	W/A 82% H/A 94%	4.4.b	virus in corneal stroma
F	2 8/12	Luhya	Perforation + secundary infection	+	W/A 61% H/A 76% RBP: 3.2 Alb 2460	4.4.c–d	
M	1 4/12	Elgeyo	Hypopyon ulcer	+	RBP: 1.9 Alb 1620	4.4.e	
F	4	Luhya	Herpetic keratitis	+	W/A 74% RBP: 2.7 Alb 3090	3.3	
F	8	Kalengin	Phlyctaenular keratitis Perforation		malnutrition	4.4.f–g	tuberculosis
F	2 6/12	Luhya	Healing corneal ulcer		?		
F	1 2/12	Luhya	Herpetic keratitis		?		
M	7/12	Luo	Corneal necrosis		W/A 77% Breast-feeding	4.4.h	
F	1 6/12	Luo	Corneal staphyloma		overfed	4.4.i	

TM: Traditional medicine was applied; W/A: Weight for Age; H/A: Height for Age; RBP: Retinol Binding Protein in serum; Alb: Albumin in serum in mg%.

group of the children in Western Province. Moreover, our patients are comparable to other published measles patients, for example the group of Gupta and Singh from Tanzania (1975).

Weight for Age	Mukumu I	Gupta-Singh
≤ 60%	5%	7%
61–80%	50%	37%
≥ 81%	45%	56%

This confirms again, that in our group the patients are generally not in a worse or better nutritional status than the general population.

b. Sample size

The possibility exists, that our sample is too small to detect a positive association, for which purpose a much larger sample might be needed. But also then, a positive outcome is − of course − not guaranteed.

The question remains however, whether all this effort would be worthwhile. In the present study no association between the nutritional status and the self-healing measles-keratitis was found.

On theoretical grounds it may be expected, that *all* children with severe Protein Energy Malnutrition have a viral measles-keratitis. This would result however in only a little higher incidence of this keratitis in severely malnourished children compared to a group of well-nourished children. This difference can therefore only be detected in a very large sample. On the overall incidence of the measles keratitis this effect is minimal.

Corneal erosions

In the electron-microscope it was shown that the corneal erosions are direct extensions of the measles-keratitis. This finding confirmed the clinical impression. Since however the measles-keratitis is independent of the nutritional status of the affected children (§6.2) the same will probably apply to the corneal erosions. The data presented in table 6.3 point in the same direction.

If these erosions play a role in the pathogenesis of Post-Measles-Blindness − and I think they do − they constitute an important corneal factor, present in at least 4% of our patients, independently of their nutritional status.

Late complications

The data regarding the nutritional status of the children with late corneal complications have only a limited value for two reasons:

(a) A sometimes considerable time has elapsed since the acute stage of the measles.

(b) These patients are most probably a very selected sample of the children with late ocular complications. Usually these complications are associated with malnutrition and therefore with a higher mortality. The children presented here, survived the measles, possibly because of a relatively good nutritional status.

In my opinion no conclusion whatsoever is to be drawn from this table.

78

7 — Discussion and Conclusion

7.1. The pathogenesis of Post-Measles-Blindness

7.1.1. Measles.

The incentive for this study was the existence of Post-Measles-Blindness: in several developing countries 1% of all children with measles sustain permanent ocular damage of corneal origin. Surprisingly, little was known about the corneal signs of early measles. In this study it was demonstrated that at least 76% of the examined measles-children had an early viral keratitis. In the following paragraphs this observation will be taken as the most logical starting point for the thinking about the etiology of Post-Measles-Blindness.

It was demonstrated that the nutritional status had no influence on the extent of this keratitis.

Our group of patients is representative for the children in Western Province and I have no reason to believe that another group of patients from this area would show this measles-keratitis to a substantially different extent.

The matter remains whether this keratitis is a peculiar finding for our group of patients, or that it is allowed to extrapolate our findings to all children with measles. There are some arguments in favour of this extrapolation, but much work is still to be done to justify this assumption.

(1) Trantas, working in Turkey (1903) found an incidence of 75% for this keratitis. The nutritional status is not mentioned.
(2) Thygeson (1959), reporting from the USA, states that probably all children have a viral epithelial keratitis in measles.
(3) Sauter (1976), reported a 30% incidence for measles-keratitis, in a cross sectional study in well-nourished children. This is comparable with 75% in a longitudinal study.

In this study it was found that this measles-keratitis — as a sign of measles — is independent from the nutritional status of the affected children. Also Thygeson's statement points in the same direction. This means that quite possibly no important differences will exist for the incidence of this keratitis in rich or developing countries.

7 out of 188 children (4%) with measles-keratitis developed central corneal erosions. For clinical reasons and because of the supporting electron microscopical findings, this is to be considered as a direct effect of the measles-keratitis, directly related to measles-virus replication in the corneal epithelial cells.

This means, that the majority of measles children, have — intrinsically to the measles infection — a cornea more open to complications. In 4% of these children even macro-erosions were found, a finding which in my opinion might play an important role in the pathogenesis of Post-Measles-Blindness. Whether the lower age at which these occur plays a role, remains to be investigated.

7.1.2. Corneal ulcers and collagenase

The development of corneal ulcers requires the breakdown of stromal collagen, by endogenous or exogenous collagenase (Itoi et al. 1969; Berman 1978). The pathogenesis of Post-Measles-Blindness must therefore probably be centered around the presence of collagenase. Pirie, Werb and Burleigh (1975) have been able to demonstrate this presence of collagenase in cases of Vitamin A dependent keratomalacia.

In measles several potential sources for collagenase might be available. Because of epithelial damage (measles, traditional medicines, bacterial or viral superinfection, Vitamin A deficiency or exposure) endogenous collagenase may be activated (Burda and Fisher 1960; Berman 1978; Van Horn et al. 1978). Another potential source of endogenous collagenase are the leucocytes, activated in cases of toxic or bacterial keratitis (Rowsey et al. 1976).

Bacterial infections easily supervene on a damaged cornea and — e.g. pseudomonas aeruginosa — can release a potent exogenous collagenase (van Horn et al. 1978). This means that in measles-keratitis several sources for collagenase might be available. Whether the pathological changes found in the keratocytes (§5.3) have any significance in this respect is unclear.

7.1.3. Malnutrition

According to common clinical opinion Post-Measles-Blindness occurs preferentially in connection with malnutrition.

The most important, dynamic, aspect of acute malnutrition is the katabolic deterioration of the metabolism. As part of the total "disadaption" especially the protein metabolism is severely disturbed: the emphasis is on a decreased synthesis of serumproteins, and a suppression of the immunesystem. Malnutrition enhances infection: in malnourished children a prolonged excretion of measles virus from the nasal mucosa was found, also (bacterial) complications are more frequent.

It was also found (Vasantha 1969) that in cases of kwashiorkor the biochemical equilibrium between the different forms of collagen in the skin shifted towards the more soluble tropocollagen. Under normal circumstances no tropocollagen is to be found in the cornea (Holt and Kinoshita 1973).

It is now very attractive to speculate, that the same mechanism might contribute to the pathogenesis of Post-Measles-Blindness: measles and its sequelae provide collagenase, whereas malnutrition brings the collagen in a more soluble state which facilitates its disintegration.

This theory could at least to some extent explain why the more severe corneal complications are connected with malnutrition. This may be an attractive hypothesis, but remains an object of much speculation.

7.1.4. Vitamin A deficiency

For some people Post-Measles-Blindness is identical to Vitamin A dependent keratomalacia. For this reason measles is frequently described as a mere trigger for the development of keratomalacia. From this study it appears however, that measles in itself might at least be an extremely important cause, because of its intrinsic and direct effects on the cornea. Also malnutrition, because of its effects on the immune system and proteinsynthesis is an undeniable factor in the pathogenesis of Post-Measles-Blindness.

From this study, no answer as to the significance of Vitamin A deficiency for the pathogenesis of PMB can be given. It must be stated however, that to dismiss measles as merely a trigger for keratomalacia does injustice to the significance of the intrinsic involvement of the cornea in measles and the possible pathogenetic implication of this observation (cfr Oomen and ten Doesschate 1973).

7.2. The prevention of Post-Measles-Blindness

The previous paragraph on the pathogenesis of Post-Measles-Blindness gives several starting points for the prevention of Post-Measles-Blindness: vaccination for the prevention of measles, topical treatment of the cornea and general measures for improvement of the nutritional status.

7.2.1. Measles vaccination

The "International Agency for the Prevention of Blindness" accepted at its first World Assembly (1978, Oxford) that measles-immunization-programmes should be developed for the prevention of anterior segment blindness, especially in Africa (IAPB 1980). Even when measles is considered only as a trigger for keratomalacia, this is an important policy statement. This recommendation of the IAPB gets however its full weight when the association between measles and the cornea is realized: in my opinion measles vaccination is mandatory (cfr Olurin 1970). To be effective the "cold chain" must be maintained from factory to patient. In Kenya this appeared possible (Lema 1975).

7.2.2. Topical treatment of the cornea

In §2.6 several possibilities for the topical treatment of corneal conditions along traditional African lines were collected. In most instances a deleterious effect of these preparations on the cornea is likely. A considerable number of cases with potential PMB will be saved from losing eyesight when these preparations are withheld.

Also in this study it was found, that treatment of the cornea with eye ointment, prevented the occurrence of early complications. It is my conviction, that this beneficial effect is primarily caused by the ointment base: the fatty base acts as a lubricant and prevents the newly formed epithelium from being scraped off: the development of erosions is avoided. Its beneficial effect in cases of (potential) exposure will be self-evident.

That the ointment contained an antibiotic, may have been coincidental:

no other ointment, apart from steroid containing preparations, was available. It might have theoretical advantages to add a collagenase-inhibitor, like CaEDTA or cysteïne (Berman 1978), to the ointment, but this is probably more of theoretical than of practical importance. The readily available, good and effective tetracycline eye ointment, which is nearly always in stock serves the purpose as well.

In conclusion: in underprevileged conditions every child with measles must be treated with topical application of eye-ointment, frequently and as long as he is ill from measles. Some traditional african eye medicines seem to be harmful and their application should be avoided.

7.2.3. Improvement of the nutritional status

It will be self-evident that children acutely ill with measles must be treated with adequate fluids, food and extra vitamins, to compensate for their deteriorated nutritional status.

Improvement of the nutritional status of the whole population, by nutrition education, improvement of horticulture and agriculture, mother and child clinics and other measures is probably the most important factor to improve "Public Health". This will also reduce the severity of measles and reduce substantially the incidence of Post-Measles-Blindness.

This is the hardest, but on the long run, the most effective way for a permanent prevention of Post-Measles-Blindness.

7.3. The measles-keratitis in immunosuppression

In cases of severe immunosuppression, when no rash develops, viral complications of measles occur, and probably also the viral measles-keratitis runs its normal course. We were able to observe at least two, markedly malnourished children, admitted because of a viral pneumonia. They had a typical measles-keratitis, but no rash was observed.

Another child, a 7 month old boy, was admitted with a classical keratomalacia, Bitot's spots in the right eye, and corneal necrosis of the left eye. Clinically no signs of a measles infection were apparent, or known to the mother. On laboratory examination however a positive anti-measles IgM was found, as proof of a recent infection.

These observations may have some practical consequences:
(a) In children with malnutrition, who contract a measles infection, the cornea is even more in danger than in well nourished children but now without the warning given by the rash.

It also offers the possibility that in cases of spontaneous keratomalacia, triggered by a feverish disease, the corneal necrosis is in fact initiated by a measles infection, undiagnosed because of the lack of a rash.

It might therefore be worthwhile to make a careful immunological study of children with "spontaneous" keratomalacia, in view a possible role of undiagnosed measles in these cases of keratomalacia.

(b) Immunosuppression can also be a consequence of the therapy for e.g. leukemia. Here also the possibility of a rashless measles infection exists. The existance of a viral conjunctivo-keratitis is then of high diagnostic value. (cfr Haltia et al. 1978).

7.4. Measles and herpes simplex keratitis

Much attention has been given to a possible connection between measles and a herpes simplex infection of the cornea.

Sauter (1976) observed in 2% of early measles a dendritic keratitis. In 480 early measles cases however, I never observed a herpetic infection. Careful slitlampexamination and the different clinical course always excluded the existence of a dendritic keratitis.

In cases with late complications the situation might be different. Two cases of herpetic keratitis — with their characteristic appearance and clinical course — were observed. It is remarkable, that both occurred a long time after the outbreak of the rash. It remains a matter of speculation in how far the use of (steroid containing?) traditional medicines in at least one case could play a role.

This observation confirms a report from Nigeria: Sandford-Smith and Whittle (1979) were able to culture the herpes virus from some corneal ulcers after measles.

In conclusion: the herpes simplex virus probably plays a role in the causation of late corneal complications.

7.5. Conclusion

The incentive for this study was the existence of Post-Measles-Blindness in developing countries: around 1% of all children with measles sustain permanent ocular damage of corneal origin.

In this first, longitudinal, study on the corneal effects of measles it was found, that the majority of our patients experienced a viral keratitis, as a sign of measles. This keratitis is independent of the nutritional status. In my opinion this keratitis is an important factor in the pathogenesis of Post-Measles-Blindness. Other important factors are malnutrition and the topical treatment given. Post-Measles-Blindness is therefore caused by an interaction of three factors: infection, malnutrition and treatment, each of which gets a different accent in individual cases. The conclusion from this study must be, that the measles infection with its effects on the cornea is much more important than is generally accepted. Moreover, more emphasis should be on what happens in the cornea: the measles infection, traditional and modern medicines, exposure.

With a little exaggeration my opinion regarding the pathogenesis of Post-Measles-Blindness can be summarized as follows: the existence of the measles-keratitis explains why Post-Measles-Blindness exists, the epidemiology of malnutrition explains why it happens in underprivileged populations.

For the prevention of Post-Measles-Blindness all factors involved in its pathogenesis should be attacked: measles vaccination, protection of the cornea with ointment, avoiding the application of some harmful traditional medicines, and improvement of the nutritional status, will all contribute their part in the reduction and eventual eradication of Post-Measles-Blindness.

References

Agarwal LP and Adhaulia HN (1954) Role of vitamin A in the healing of corneal ulcers. Ophthalmologica 128, 6–14

Agarwal LP and Malhoutra RL (1955) Conjunctival smear cytology in xerosis. Ophthalmologica 130, 378–386

Allansmith, M and Hutchison D (1967) Immunoglobulins in the conjunctiva. Immunology 12, 225–229

Allansmith MR, Whitney CR, McClellan, BH and Newman LP (1973) Immunoglobulins in the human eye. Location, type and amount. Arch Ophthal 89, 36–45

Allansmith MR and McClellan BH (1975) Immunoglobulins in the human cornea. Amer J Ophthal 80, 123–132

Alleyne GAO, Hay RW, Picou DI, Stanfield JP and Whitehead RG (1977) Protein-energy malnutrition. London, Edward Arnold

Amies CR, Loewenthal LJA, Murray NL and Scott GJ (1953) Blindness in the Bantu. A survey of external eye disease and malnutrition in the North Eastern Transvaal. South Afr Med J 27, 593–597

Animashaun A (1977) Measles and blindness in Nigerian children. Nigerian J Pediat 4, 10–13

Armengaud M, Frament V, Biram D and Mar ID (1961) Les kératites de la rougeole en milieu africain à Dakar. Bull Soc Méd Afr noire de Langue fr 6, 36–44

Aronson SB, Yamamoto EA, Enterline ML and Bedford MJ (1967) Mechanisms of the host response in the eye. Arch Ophth 78, 384–396

Arroyave G and Calcaño M (1979) Descenso de los niveles séricos de retinol y de su proteína de enlace (RBP) durante las infecciones. Arch Latinoamer Nutr 29, 233–260

Arroyave G, Viteri F, Béhar M and Scrimshaw NS (1959) Impairment of intestinal absorption of vitamin A palmitate in severe protein malnutrition (Kwashiorkor). Amer J Clin Nutr 7, 185–190

Arroyave G, Wilson D, Méndez J, Béhar M and Scrimshaw NS (1961) Serum and liver vitamin A and lipids in children with severe protein malnutrition. Amer J Clin Nutr 9, 180–185

Attal C and Mozziconacci P (1970) Measles, Clinical features. In: Debré R and Celers J (eds) Clinical Virology, the evaluation and management of human viral diseases. WB Saunders, Philadelphia, London, Toronto

Axton JHM (1979) Measles and the state of nutrition. SA Med Tydskrif 55, 125–126

Ayanru JO (1974) Blindness in the midwestern state of Nigeria. Trop Geogr Med 26, 325–332

Ayanru JO (1978) Affections of conjunctiva and cornea in Bendel State of Nigeria. Trop Geogr Med 30, 69

Azizi A and Krakovsky D (1965) Keratoconjunctivitis as a constant sign of measles. Ann paediat 204, 397–405

Baghdassarian SA and Tabbara KF (1975) Childhood blindness in Lebanon. Amer J Ophthal 79, 827–830

Bailey KV (1975) Malnutrition in the African region. WHO Chronicle 29, 354–364

Baisya DC, Dutta LC, Goswami P and Saha SK (1971) Role of serum protein in the ocular manifestations of vitamin A deficiency. Brit J Ophthal 55, 700–703

Bakker A (1940) Klinische und experimentelle Untersuchungen über Augenverletzungen durch Saponin. Ophthalmologica 99, 356–366

Bauer F (1970) Über den Verlauf immunbiologischer Vorgänge in der Hornhaut. Klin Mbl Augenheilk 157, 230–233

Bech V (1959) Studies on the development of complement fixing antibodies in measles patients. J Immunol 83, 267–275

Beaver DL (1961) Vitamin A deficiency in the germ-free rat. Amer J Pathol 38, 335–357

Benezra D and Chirambo MC (1977) Incidence and causes of blindness among the under 5 age group in Malawi. Brit J Ophthal 61, 154–157

Benezra D and Chirambo MC (1978) Childhood blindness in a developing country. Metabol Ophthal 2, 103–105

Berman M (1978) Regulation of collagenase. Therapeutic considerations. Trans Ophthal Soc UK 98, 397–405

Berman MB, Barber JC, Talamo RC and Langley CE (1973) Corneal ulceration and the serum antiproteases. Invest Ophthal 12, 759–770

Berman M, Dohlman CH, Gnädinger M and Davison P (1971) Characterization of collagenolytic activity in the ulcerating cornea. Exp Eye Res 11, 255–257

Berman M, Leary R and Gage J (1977) Latent collagenase in the ulcerating rabbit cornea. Exp Eye Res 25, 435–445

Berman MB and Manabe R (1973) Corneal collagenases: evidence for zinc metallo-enzymes. Annals Ophthal 5, 1193–1209

Bietti G (1977) Ocular manifestations of vitamin deficiencies and disordered vitamin metabolism. Metabol Ophthal 1, 81–89

Bisley GG (1963) The prevention and treatment of blindness in Kenya. East Afr Med J 40, 570–573

Blackfan KD and Wolbach SB (1933) Vitamin A deficiency in infants. J Pediat 3, 679–706

Blatz G (1956) Hornhauteinschmelzung nach Masern. Klin Mbl Augenheilk 129, 762–772

Bloch CE (1921) Clinical investigation of xerophthalmia and dystrophy in infants and young children (Xerophthalmia et dystrophia alipogenetica). J Hygiene 19, 283–307

Blumenthal CJ (1950) Malnutritional keratoconjunctivitis. South Afr Med J 24, 191–198

Blumenthal CJ (1954) Blindness and malnutrition in the Eastern Cape Province. South Afr Med J 28, 967–971

Blumenthal CJ (1960) Malnutritional keratitis. Proc Nutrit Soc 19, 92–105

Bohigian G, Valenton M, Okumoto M and Caraway MBL (1974) Collagenase inhibitors in Pseudomonas keratitis. Arch Ophthal 91, 52–56

Bonamour G (1953) La participation de la cornée à l'éruption cutanée de la face au cours des maladies infectieuses éruptives de l'enfance: rougeole et scarlatine. Bull Soc Ophtal 82, 95–97

Bonamour G (1953) Les manifestations oculaires des maladies infectieuses éruptives de l'enfance. J Méd Lyon 34, 557–567

Brown SI, Akiya S and Weller CA (1969) Prevention of the ulcers of the alkali-burned cornea. Arch Opthal 82, 95–97

Brown SI, Bloomfield SE and Tam WI (1974) The cornea-destroying enzyme of Pseudomonas aeruginosa. Invest Opthal 13, 174–180

Brown SI and Weller CA (1970) The pathogenesis and treatment of collagenase-induced diseases of the cornea. Trans Amer Acad Ophthal Otolaryng 74, 375–393

Brown SI, Weller CA and Wassermann HE (1969) Collagenolytic activity of alkali-burned corneas, Arch Ophthal 81, 370–373

Bücklers M (1969) Erblindung bei Masern mit nachfolgender Pigmententartung der Netzhaut. Ophthalmologica 159, 274–294

Burda CD and Fisher E (1960) Corneal destruction by extracts of cephalosporium mycelium. Amer J Ophthal 50, 926–937

Burkitt WR (1975) Suggestions for the development of rural eye services in Africa. Trop Doctor 5, 30–32

Burnet FM (1968) Measles as an index of immunological function. Lancet II, 610–613

Buschke W (1949) Experimentelle Studien zur Patho-physiologie des Hornhautepithels: Zell-Bewegungen bei der Wundheilung, Zell-Teilung, Mitosehemmung und andere Kernphänomene. Ophthalmologica 118, 407–439

Bwibo NO (1970) Measles in Uganda. An analysis of children with measles admitted to Mulago hospital. Trop Geogr Med 22, 167–171

Calcott RD (1956) Blindness in Kenya. British Empire Society for the Blind, London

Carlström G (1962) Relation of measles to other viruses. Amer J Dis Child 103, 287–291

Carter-Dawson L, Tanaka M, Kuwabara T and Bieri JG (1980) Early corneal changes in Vitamin A deficient rats. Exp Eye Res 30, 261–268

Casanovas J (1976) Keratite ponctuee superficielle. Ann d'Oculist 209, 379–382

Chi HH, Teng CC and Katzin HM (1960) Healing process in the mechanical denudation of the corneal endothelium. Amer J Ophthal 49, 693–703

Chirambo MC and Benezra D (1976) Causes of blindness among students in blind school institutions in a developing country. Brit J Ophthal 60, 665–668

Choudhury MI (1976) Incidence and causes of blindness amongst the rural population. Bangladesh Med Res Counc Bull 2, 71–74

Chown B (1939) Giant cell pneumonia of infancy as a manifestation of vitamin A deficiency. Amer J Dis Child 57, 489–505

Clercq E de and Merigan TC (1970) Current concepts of interferon and interferon induction. Ann Rev Med 21, 17–46

Cooper WC, Good RA and Mariani T (1974) Effects of protein insufficiency on immune responsiveness. Amer J Clin Nutr 27, 647–664

Coovadia HM, Brain P, Hallett AF, Wesley A, Henderson LG and Vos GH (1977) Immunoparesis and outcome in measles. Lancet 1, 619–621

Coovadia HM, Wesley A and Brain P (1978) Immunological events in acute measles influencing outcome. Arch Dis Childh 53, 861–867

Corcelle M and Cloix C (1961) Les kératites des comateux. Ann d'Oculist 194, 199–210

Cordero-Moreno R (1973) Etiological factors in tropical eye diseases. Am J Ophthal 75, 349–364

Cosmettatos GF (1908) Des complications cornéennes de la rougeole. Arch d'Ophtal 28, 299–306

Crowder JI and Sexton RR (1964) Keratoconjunctivitis resulting from the sap of candelebra cactus and the pencil tree. Amer J Ophthal 72, 476–484

Cruickshank R, Duguid JP, Marmion BP and Swain RHA (1974) Medical microbiology; 12ed. Volume 1: Microbial infections. Edinburgh, English Language Book Society and Churchill Livingstone

Cruickshank R, Standard KL and Russell HBL (1976) Epidemiology and community health in warm climate countries. Edinburgh, Churchill Livingstone

Czajkowski J and Heneen WK (1976) Electron microscopy of mitotic cells in a measles-carrier human cell line. Hereditas 83, 257–264

Damiean-Gillet M (1958) Conjunctival lesions in avitaminosis A. A histopathological study. Trop Geogr Med 10, 233–238

Darby WJ, McGanity WJ, McLaren DS, Paton D, Alemu AZ and Medhen, AMG (1960) Bitot's spots and vitamin A deficiency. Publ Hlth Rep 75, 738–743

Davison PF and Berman M (1973) Corneal collagenase: specific cleavage of types $(\alpha 1)_2 \alpha 2$ and $(\alpha 1)_3$ collagens. Conn Tissue Res 2, 57–64

Dawson CR (1976) How does the external eye resist infection? Editorial. Invest Ophthal 15, 971–974

Doesschate J ten (1968) Causes of blindness in and around Surabaja, East Java, Indonesia. Thesis Djakarta. Djakarta, Oleh

Dohlman CH (1971) The function of the corneal epithelium in health and disease. Invest Ophthal 10, 383–407

Dohlman CH and Kalevar V (1972) Cornea in hypovitaminosis A and protein deficiency. Israël J Med Sci 8, 1179–1183

O'Donovan C (1971) Measles in Kenyan children. East Afr Med J 48, 526–532

Donshik PC, Berman MB, Dohlman CH, Gage J and Rose J (1978) Effect of topical corticosteroids on ulceration in alkali-burned corneas. Arch Ophthal 96, 2117–2120

Dossetor J, Whittle HC and Greenwood BM (1977) Persistent measles infection in malnourished children. Brit med J 1, 1633–1635

Dubos RJ and Schaedler RW (1958) Effect of dietary proteins and amino acids on the susceptibility of mice to bacterial infections. J Exp Med 108, 69–81

Dugdale AE (1971) An age-independent anthropometric index of nutritional status. Amer J Clin Nutr 24, 174–176

Duke-Elder S (1965) System of ophthalmology, Volume VIII: Diseases of the conjunctiva and associated diseases of the corneal epithelium. Henry Kimpton, London

Duke-Elder S and MacFaul PA (1972) In: Duke-Elder S, System of Ophthalmology, Volume XIV: Injuries. Henry Kimpton, London

Eddy TP (1977) An error of medicine? Kwashiorkor and the "protein gap". Trop Doctor 7, 28−32

Edelman R, Suskind R, Olson RE and Sirisinha S (1973) Mechanisms of defective delayed cutaneous hypersensitivity in children with protein-calorie malnutrition. Lancet I, 506−508

Editorial (1973) Pathogenesis of Measles. Brit Med J 2, 187−188

Editorial (1976) Pulmonary complications of measles. Brit med J 2, 777−778

Editorial (1976) Measles in the tropics. Brit med J 2, 1339−1340

Eleftheriou D-S and Djacos C (1950) Lésions anatomo-pathologiques de la cornée dans les oedèmes de carence. Arch d'Ophtal 10, 217−227

Emiru VP (1971) The cornea in Kwashiorkor. J Trop Pediat Child Hlth 17, 118−134

Emran N and Sommer A (1979) Lissamine Green staining in the clinical diagnosis of xerophthalmia. Arch Ophthal 97, 2333−2335

Enders JF, McCarthy K, Mitus A and Cheatham WJ (1959) Isolation of measles virus at autopsy in cases of giant-cell pneumonia without rash. New Engl J Med 261, 875−881

Eppenstein A (1918) Neuritis optici und Iridozyklitis infolge von Masern. Klin Mbl Augenheilk 60, 245−248

Eubank MD (1964) Differential diagnosis of viral keratitis. Amer J Ophthal 58, 300−301

Fedukowicz HB (1978) External infections of the eye. p 214−217 2nd ed. New York, Appleton

Fell HB (1965) The effect of vitamin A on the breakdown and synthesis of intercellular material in skeletal tissue in organ culture. Proc Nutr Soc 24, 166−170

Fischer JN (1846) Eigenthümliche Zerstörung der Hornhaut in Folge unterdrückter Masern. In: Lehrbuch der gesammten Entzündungen und organischen Krankheiten des menschlichen Auges. p 275. Prag, Borrosch and André

Fisher E and Allen JH (1958) Corneal ulcers produced by cell-free extracts of pseudomonas aeruginosa. Amer J Ophthal 46, 21−27

Fisher E and Allen JH (1958) Mechanism of corneal destruction by pseudomonas proteases. Amer J Ophthal 46, 249−255

Fleury H and Pasquier P du (1977) Replication of measles virus in a cell culture from a glioblastoma of human origin. J Neuro Exp Neurol, 842−845

Florman AL and Agatston HJ (1962) Keratoconjunctivitis as a diagnostic aid in measles. JAMA 179, 568−570

Fogle JA, Kenyon KR, Stark WJ and Green WR (1975) Defective epithelial adhesion in anterior corneal dystrophies. Amer J Ophthal 79, 925−940

Forbes CE and Scheifele DW (1973) The management of measles in Nairobi. East Afr Med J 50, 159−168

François J (1978) Erosion dystrophique récidivante de l'épithélium cornéen. Ophthalmologica 177, 121−133

Franken S (1974) Measles and xerophthalmia in East Africa. Trop Geogr Med 26, 39−44

Fraser GR (1968) The causes of severe visual handicap among schoolchildren in South Australia. Med J Austr 1, 615−620

Fraser GR and Friedmann AI (1967) The causes of blindness in childhood. Baltimore, Johns Hopkins Press

Frederique G, Howard RO and Boniuk V (1969) Corneal ulcers in rubeola. Amer J Ophthal 68, 996−1003

Freedman J (1973) Survey of ocular disease among the Nama people of South West Africa. Brit J Ophthal 57, 681−687

Friedenwald JS, Buschke W and Morris ME (1945) Mitotic activity and wound healing in the corneal epithelium of vitamin A deficient rats. J Nutrition 29, 299−308

Frood JDL, Whitehead RG and Coward WA (1971) Relationship between pattern of infection and development of hypoalbuminaemia and hypo-β-lipoproteinaemia in rural Ugandan children. Lancet I, 1047−1049

Fuchs E (1893) Lehrbuch der Augenheilkunde; 3e dr. Leipzig, Deuticke

Fulton RE and Middleton PJ (1975) Immunofluorescence in diagnosis of measles infections in children. J Pediatrics 86, 17−22

Garrow JS and Pike MC (1967) The short-term prognosis of severe primary infantile malnutrition. Brit J Nutr 21, 155−165

Gaud F (1958) Les complications oculaires des maladies infectieuses éruptives de l'enfance. Arch d'Ophtal 18, 25−56

Geddes TD and Gregory WJ (1974) Transferrin, immunoglobulins and prognosis in measles in the tropics. Trop Geogr Med 26, 79–83

Gemert W, Valkenburg HA and Muller AS (1977) Agents affecting health of mother and child in a rural area of Kenya. II. The diagnosis of measles under field conditions. Trop Geogr Med 29, 303–313

Germuth Jr FG, Maumenee AE, Senterfit LB and Pollack AD (1962) Immunohistologic studies on antigen-antibody reactions in the avascular cornea. I. Reactions in rabbits actively sensitized to foreign protein. J Exp Med 115, 919–931

Glover J and Walker RJ (1964) Absorption and transport of vitamin A. Exp Eye Res 3, 327–348

Gnädinger MC, Itoi M, Slansky HH and Dohlman CH (1969) The role of collagenase in the alkali-burned cornea. Amer J Ophthal 68, 478–483

Golden MHN, Patrick J, Jackson AA and Picou DI (1975) Serum-albumin in oedematous malnutrition. Lancet 2, 1044

Goldstein H (1976) Incidence, prevalence and causes of blindness in selected countries. III. United States, Africa, America, Oceania. Publ Health Reviews 5, 35–66

Gopalan C, Venkatachalam PS and Bhavani B (1960) Studies of vitamin A deficiency in children. Amer J Clin Nutr 8, 833–840

Government of Kenya (1970) National Atlas of Kenya, Survey of Kenya, 3d ed. Government Press, Nairobi

Government of Kenya (1973) Kenya, an official handbook. East African Publishing house

Government of Kenya (1977) Ministry of Finance and Planning. The Rural Kenyan Nutrition Survey. In: "Social perspectives".

Grana PC (1946) Conjunctivitis and dermatitis due to "Beach apple". Arch Ophthal 35, 421–422

Grayson M (1979) Diseases of the cornea. CV Mosby, St Louis, Toronto, London

Grimble RF and Whitehead RG (1970) Fasting serum-aminoacid patterns in Kwashiorkor and after administration of different levels of protein. Lancet I, 918–920

Grist NR (1950) The pathogenesis of measles: review of the literature and discussion of the problem. Glasgow Med J 31, 431–441

Gross J and Nagai Y (1965) Specific degradation of the collagen molecule by tadpole collagenolytic enzyme. Proc NAS 54, 1197–1204

Gupta BM and Singh M (1975) Mortality and morbidity pattern in measles in Tanga District, Tanzania. Trop geogr Med 27, 383–386

Haas JH de, Posthuma JH and Meulemans O (1941) Xerophthalmia in children in Batavia. Indian J Pediat 8, 139–157

Hall WW and Martin SJ (1975) The structural proteins of measles virus. In: Negative strand viruses; ed. by BJ Mahy and RD Barry, p 89–103. New York, Academic Press

Haltia M, Tarkkanen A, Vaheri A, Paetau A, Kaakinen K and Erkkilä H (1978) Measles retinopathy during immunosuppression. Brit J Ophthal 62, 356–360

Hanna C, Fraunfelder FT, Cable M and Hardberger RE (1973) The effect of ophthalmic ointments on corneal wound healing. Amer J Ophthal 76, 193–200

Harley RD (ed)(1975) Pediatric Ophthalmology, WB Saunders, Philadelphia, London, Toronto

Hartmann K (1940) Augenschädigung durch den Saft der Euphorbia Peplus (Wolfsmilch). Klin Mbl Augenheilk 104, 324–326

Hay RW, Whitehead RG and Spicer CC (1975) Serum-albumin as a prognostic indicator in oedematous malnutrition. Lancet 2, 427–429

Haydn M (1970) Erblindung beider Augen nach Masernerkrankung. Klin Mbl Augenheilk 156, 539–543

Hendrickse RG (1975) Problems of future measles vaccination in developing countries. Trans Roy Soc Trop Med Hyg 69, 31–34

Henkind P and Friedman AH (1971) External ocular pigmentation. Int Opthal Clinics 11, 87–111

Herrman C (1914) Measles: Incubation, infectivity, immunity, early manifestations. Arch Pediat 31, 885–894

Hiro Y and Yamada M (1936) Die Masern und die Ceratomalacie. Mschr Kinderheilk 65, 439–445

Hodge AJ and Schmitt FO (1960) The charge profile of the tropocollagen macro-molecule and the packing arrangement in native-type collagen fibrils. Proc NAS 46, 186–197

Holmes WJ (1959) Geographic ophthalmology. Asia, Australia, and Africa. Springfield, Thomas

Holt WS and Kinoshita JH (1973) The soluble proteins of the bovine cornea. Invest Ophthal 12, 114–126

Hook CW, Brown SI, Iwanij W and Nakanishi I (1971) Characterization and inhibition of corneal collagenase. Invest Ophthal 10, 496–503

Horn DL van, Davis SD, Hyndiuk RA and Alpren TVP (1978) Pathogenesis of experimental pseudomonas keratitis in the guinea pig: bacteriologic, clinical, and microscopic observations. Invest Ophthal 17, 1076–1086

Horn DL van, Schultz RO and Kwasny GP (1973) Pseudomonas corneal ulceration: an electronic microscopic study. Annals Ophthal 5, 1183–1188

Horn DL van, Schutten WH, Hyndiuk RA and Kurz P (1980) Xerophthalmia in Vitamin A deficient rabbits. Clinical and ultrastructural alterations in the cornea. Invest Ophthal 19, 1067–1079

Imperato PJ (1975) Traditional medical practitioners among the Bambara of Mali and their role in the modern health care delivery system. Trop Geogr Med 27, 211–221

Imperato PJ and Traoré D (1969) Traditional beliefs about measles and its treatment among the Bambara of Mali. Trop Geogr Med 21, 62–67

Ingenbleek Y, Schrieck HG van den, Nayer Ph de and Visscher M de (1975) The role of retinol-binding protein in protein-calorie malnutrition. Metabolism 24, 633–641

Ingenbleek Y, Schrieck HG van den, Nayer Ph de and Visscher M de (1975) Albumin, transferrin and the thyroxine-binding prealbumin/retinol-binding protein (TBPA-RBP) complex in assessment of malnutrition. Clin Chim Acta 63, 61–67

Ingenbleek Y, Visscher M de and Nayer Ph de (1972) Measurement of prealbumin as index of protein-calorie malnutrition. Lancet 2, 106–108

International Agency for the Prevention of Blindness (1980) World Blindness and its prevention. Oxford University Press, Oxford, New York, Toronto

Itoi M, Gnädinger MC, Slansky HH and Dohlman CH (1969) Prévention d'ulcères du stroma de la cornée grâce à l'utilisation d'un sel de calcium d'EDTA. Arch d'Ophtal 29, 389–392

Itoi M, Gnädinger MC, Slansky HH, Freeman MI and Dohlman CH (1969) Collagenase in the cornea. Exp Eye Res 8, 369–373

Iverson HA (1964) Survey of eye diseases in Uganda. East Afr Med J 41, 289–294

Jamieson SW (1970) Eye survey – Mrewa Trust Lands. Postgrad Med J 46, 557–561

Jansen AAJ and Bailey KV (1972) The early detection of childhood malnutrition in the South Pacific. WHO Report 5601

Jelliffe DB (1974) Child health in the tropics; 4 ed. Bristol, Western Printing Services

Jones BR (1958) The clinical features of viral keratitis and a concept of their pathogenesis. Proc Royal Soc Med 51, 13–20

Jones BR (1960) The differential diagnosis of punctate keratitis. Trans Ophthal Soc UK 80, 665–675

Kallman F, Adams JM, Williams RC and Imagawa DI (1959) Fine structure of cellular inclusions in measles virus infections. J Biophys Biochem Cytol 6, 379–382

Kaufman HE (1960) The diagnosis of corneal herpes simplex infection by fluorescent antibody staining. Arch Ophthal 64, 382–384

Kenyon KR, Berman M, Rose J and Gage J (1979) Prevention of stromal ulceration in the alkali-burned rabbit cornea by glued-on contact lens. Evidence for the role of polymorphonuclear leukocytes in collagen degradation. Invest. Ophthalmol Visual Sci 18, 570–587

Kerby CE (1958) Causes of blindness in children of school age. Sight Sav Rev 28, 10–21

Kerharo J and Bouquet A (1948) Sur un traitement africain de différentes affections oculaires. Comptes rendus hebdomadaires des Séances de l'Academie des Sciences. Paris 226, 359–361

Kessler E, Kennah HE and Brown SI (1977) Pseudomonas protease. Purification, partial characterization, and its effect on collagen, proteoglycan, and rabbit corneas. Invest Ophthal 16, 488–497

Khodadoust AA, Silverstein AM, Kenyon KR and Dowling JE (1968) Adhesion of regenerating corneal epithelium. Amer J Ophthal 65, 339–348

Kietzman B (1968) Endophthalmitis in Nigerian children. Amer J Ophthal 65, 211–220

Kimati VP and Lyaruu B (1976) Measles complications as seen at Mwanza regional consultant and teaching hospital in 1973. East Afr Med J 53, 332–340

Kimura A, Tosaka K and Nakao T (1975) Measles rash. I. Light and electron microscopic study of skin eruptions. Arch Virol 47, 295–307

King MH (1966) Medical care in developing countries. A symposium from Makerere. Nairobi, Oxford University Press

King MH, King FMA, Morley DC, Burgess HJL and Burgess AP (1972) Nutrition for developing countries. Oxford University Press, Nairobi, London

Kinnear Brown JA (1956) Observations on the general incidence of blindness and certain other diseases in Uganda. East Afr Med J 33, 19–24

Klöne W, Kulemann H, Ward EN and Salk JE (1963) Some observations on measles induced giant cell formation. Exp Cell Res 31, 438–440

Kokwaro JO (1976) Medicinal plants in East Africa. Kampala, East African Literature Bureau

Korte R and Wiersinga A (1972) Deficiency in male prisoners reflecting borderline vitamin A intake in the population of Kenya. Trop Geogr Med 24, 339–343

Kronning E (1954) Conjunctival and corneal stainability with bengal rose. Amer J Ophthal 38, 351–361

Kuming BS (1967) The evolution of keratomalacia. Trans Ophthal Soc UK 87, 305–315

Kuming BS and Politzer WM (1967) Xerophthalmia and protein malnutrition in Bantu children. Brit J Ophthal 51, 649–666

Kusin JA, Parlindungan Sinaga HSR and Marpaung AM (1977) Xerophthalmia in North Sumatra. Trop Geogr Med 29, 41–46

Kusin JA, Soewondo W and Parlindungan Sinaga HSR (1979) Rose Bengal and Lissamine Green vital stains: useful diagnostic aids for early stages of xerophthalmia? Am J Clin Nutr 32, 1559–1561

Lagraulet J and Bard J (1967) Lésions oculaires de la rougeole dans les milieux ruraux en Afrique noire. Bull Soc Path Exot 60, 203–205

Landy D (ed)(1977) Culture, disease and healing. Studies in medical anthropology. Macmillan, New York

Lansche RK (1965) Vital staining in normal eyes and in keratoconjunctivitis sicca. Amer J Ophthal 60, 520–525

Latkovic S and Nilsson SEG (1979) The ultrastructure of the normal conjunctival epithelium of the guinea pig. I. The basal and intermediate layers of the perilimbal zone. Acta Ophthal 57, 106–122

Latkovic S and Nilsson SEG (1979) The ultrastructure of the normal conjunctival epithelium of the guinea pig. II. The superficial layer of the perilimbal zone. Acta Ophthal 57, 123–135

Latkovic S (1979) The ultrastructure of the normal conjunctival epithelium of the guinea pig. III. The bulbar zone, the zone of the fornix and the supranodular zone. Acta Ophthal 57, 305–320

Latkovic S (1979) The ultrastructure of the normal conjunctival epithelium of the guinea pig. IV. The palpebral and the perimarginal zones. Acta Ophthal 57, 321–335

Leary PM and Obst D (1966) The pattern of measles among Africans in a Bantu reserve. South Afr Med J 40, 293–295

Lema JT (1975) Three years of measles vaccination in Mombasa district – Kenya. East Afr Med J 52, 70–75

Lemp MA, Dohlman CH, Kuwabara T, Holly FJ and Carroll JM (1971) Dry eye secondary to mucus deficiency. Tr Am Acad Opth and Otol 75, 1223–1227

Lemp MA, Holly FJ, Iwata S and Dohlman CH (1970) The precorneal tear film. I. Factors in spreading and maintaining a continuous tear film over the corneal surface. Arch Ophthal 83, 89–94

Leopold IH (1973) The role of lymphocyte (cell-mediated) immunity in ocular disease. Amer J Ophthal 76, 619–631

Levenson JE (1973) The effect of short-term drying on the surface ultrastructure of the rabbit cornea: A scanning electron microscopic study. Annals Ophthal 5, 865–877

Lewis WH and Elvin-Lewis MPF (1977) Medical botany. Plants affecting man's health. New York, John Wiley

Lindstedt E (1969) Causes of blindness in Sweden. Copenhagen, Munksgaard. Acta Ophthalmologica, supplement 104

Lorenz E and Rossipal E (1965) Zur Frage der Resistenzverminderung bei Masern. Mschr Kinderheilk 113, 161–162

Lucas K (1978) Interaction of measles virus and lymphocytes. Relation to virus persistence and immunopathology. Thesis, Amsterdam. Amsterdam, Spruijt

McGlashan ND (1969) Measles, malnutrition and blindness in Luapula province, Zambia. Trop Geogr Med 21, 157–162

MacIntyre EH and Armstrong JA (1976) Fine structural changes in human astrocyte carrier lines for measles virus. Nature 263, 232–234

Mackaness GB (1971) Resistance to intracellular infection. J Infect Dis 123, 439–445

McLaren DS (1956) A study of the factors underlying the special incidence of keratomalacia in Oriya children in the Phulbani and Ganjam districts of Orissa, India. J Trop Ped 2, 135–140

McLaren DS (1959) Influence of protein deficiency and sex on the development of ocular lesions and survival time of the vitamin A-deficient rat. Brit J Ophthal 43, 234–241

McLaren DS (1960) Nutrition and eye disease in East Africa: experience in Lake and Central Provinces, Tanganyika. J Trop Med Hyg 63, 101–122

McLaren DS (1960) Malnutrition and eye disease in Tanganyika. Proc Nutr Soc 19, 89–91

McLaren DS (1963) Malnutrition and the eye. Academic Press, New York–London

McLaren DS (1966) Present knowledge of the role of vitamin A in health and disease. Trans Roy Soc Trop Med Hyg 60, 436–455

McLaren DS, Oomen HAPC and Escapini H (1966) Ocular manifestations of vitamin-A deficiency in man. Bull Wld Hlth Org 34, 357–361

McLaren DS, Pellett PL and Read WWC (1967) A simple scoring system for classifying the severe forms of protein-calorie malnutrition of early childhood. Lancet I, 533–535

McLaren DS, Faris R and Zekian B (1968) The liver during recovery from protein-calorie malnutrition. J Trop Med Hyg 71, 271–281

McLaren DS (1970) Corneal ulcers in rubeola. Letter to the Editor. Amer J Ophthal 70, 442–443

McLaren DS (1971) Classification of protein-calorie malnutrition. Lancet II, 1208

McLaren DS (1974) The great protein fiasco. Lancet II, 93–96

McLaren DS and Read WWC (1975) Weight/length classification of nutritional status. Lancet II, 219–221

MacManus EP (1968) Xerophthalmia in Matabeleland. Centr Afr J Med 14, 166–170

McPherson HJ (1954) Hypopyon corneal ulcer in Malaya. Med J Malaya 8, 318–329

Maina-Ahlberg B (1979) Agents affecting health of mother and child in a rural area of Kenya. XII: Beliefs and practices concerning treatment of measles and acute diarrhoea among the Akamba. Trop Geogr Med 31, 139–148

Manen JG van (1938) Bestrijding der blindheid in Nederlandsch Oost-Indië. Eén jaar reizend oogarts. Geneesk Ts N-Indië 78, 1724–1784

Marquardt R (1978) Allgemeine Klinik der Konjunktivitis. Klin Mbl Augenheilk 172, 799–806

Medical Research Council (1977) Clinical trial of live measles vaccine given alone and live vaccine preceded by killed vaccine. Lancet I, 571–575

Meuwissen SGM (1968) Mazelen in Afrika. Ned T Geneesk 112, 1963

Mishima S (1965) Some physiological aspects of the precorneal tear film. Arch Ophthal 73, 233–241

Mitus A, Enders JF, Craig JM and Holloway A (1959) Persistence of measles virus and depression of antibody formation in patients with giant-cell pneumonia after measles. New Engl J Med 261, 882–889

Moore Th (1957) Vitamin A. Amsterdam, Elsevier

Morgan EM and Rapp F (1977) Measles virus and its associated diseases. Bacteriol. Reviews 41, 636–666

Morley DC (1962) Measles in Nigeria. Amer J Dis Child 103, 230–233

Morley D, Woodland M and Martin WJ (1963) Measles in Nigerian children. J Hyg 61, 115–134

Morley DC, Martin WJ and Allen I (1967) Measles in East and Central Africa. East Afr Med J 44, 497–508

Morley D (1969) Severe measles in the tropics. I. Brit med J 1, 297–300

Morley D (1969) Severe measles in the tropics. II. Brit med J 1, 363–365

Morley D (1976) Paediatric priorities in evolving community programmes for developing countries. Lancet II, 1012–1014

Mortada A, Hegazy MA, Hegazy MR and Helal M (1976) The use of aloe extracts in the treatment of experimental corneal ulcers. EGY-CESK OFTALMOL 32, 424–427

Motohashi T, Nakagawa H and Okada T (1969) Fluorescent antibody technic in diagnosis of canine distemper. Veterinary Med, 1057–1060

Mueller FO (1971) Weltblindheit. Klin Mbl Augenheilk 159, 248–252

Müller W, Köhler U, Priegnitz F and Sprössig M (1967) Virusnachweis bei Erkrankung von Hornhaut und Bindehaut. Klin Mbl Augenheilk 150, 529–534

Muller AS, Voorhoeve AM, Mannetje W 't and Schulpen TWJ (1977) The impact of measles in a rural area of Kenya. East Afr Med J 54, 364–372

Muller AS, Ouma JH, Mburu FM, Blok PG and Kleevens JWL (1977) Agents affecting health of mother and child in a rural area of Kenya. I. Introduction: study design and methodology. Trop Geogr Med 29, 291–302

Muller AS (1979) Epidemiologisch onderzoek in een ontwikkelingsland. Het Machakosproject in Kenia. Med Contact nr 4, 110–112

Murray MJ and Murray AB (1977) Starvation suppression and refeeding activation of infection. An ecological necessity? Lancet I, 123–125

Muto Y, Smith JE, Milch PO and Goodman DS (1972) Regulation of retinol-binding protein metabolism by vitamin A status in the rat. J Biol Chem 247, 2542–2550

Nakai M and Imagawa DT (1969) Electron microscopy of measles virus replication. J Virology 3, 187–197

Nanagas PJ (1953) Nutritional dystrophy of corneal epithelium. Arch Ophthal 49, 536–552

Nanagas PJ (1954) Nutritional dystrophy of the corneal epithelium. Arch Ophthal 51, 456–466

Nasemann Th (1974) Viruskrankheiten der Haut, der Schleimhaut und des Genitales. Georg Thieme Verlag, Stuttgart

Nataf R, Lépine P and Bonamour G (1960) Oeil et virus, p 734–742. Paris, Masson

Nommensen FE and Dekkers NWHM (in preparation) Detection of measles antigen in conjunctival epithelial lesions staining by Lissamine Green during measles virus infection. J Med Virology

Norn MS (1964) Specific double vital staining of the cornea and conjunctiva with rose bengal and alcian blue. Acta Ophthal 42, 84–96

Norn MS (1970) Rose bengal vital staining. Staining of cornea and conjunctiva by 10% Rose Bengal, compared with 1%. Acta Ophthal 48, 546–559

Norn MS (1973) Lissamine green. Vital staining of cornea and conjunctiva. Acta Ophthal 51, 483–491

Norn MS and Opauszki A (1977) Effects of ophthalmic vehicles on the stability of the precorneal film. Acta Ophthal 55, 23–33

Norrby E (1972) Intracellular accumulation of measles virus nucleocapsid and envelope antigens. Microbios 5, 31–40

Oduori ML (1973) Practical aspects of paediatric practice in Kenya with special reference to rural paediatrics. East Afr Med J 50, 546–554

Olding-Stenkvist E and Bjorvatn B (1976) Rapid detection of measles virus in skin rashes by immunofluorescence. J Infect Dis 134, 463–469

Olurin O (1970) Etiology of blindness in Nigerian children. Amer J Ophthal 70, 533–540

Olurin O (1973) Causes of enucleation in Nigeria. Amer J Ophthal 76, 987–991

Oomen HAPC (1961) An outline of xerophthalmia. Intern Rev Trop Med 1, 131–213

Oomen HAPC (1969) Clinical epidemiology of xerophthalmia in man. Amer J Clin aspects of hypovitaminosis A. Trop Geogr Med 4, 271–315

Oomen HAPC (1969) Clinical epidemiology of xerophthalmia in man. Amer J Clin Nutr 22, 1098–1105

Oomen HAPC (1972) Xerophthalmia and hypovitaminosis A. Trop Doctor 2, 163–169

Oomen HAPC and Doesschate J ten (1973) The periodicity of xerophthalmia in South and East Asia. Ecol Food Nutr 2, 207–217

Oomen JMV (1971) Xerophthalmia in Northern Nigeria. Trop Geogr Med 23, 246–249

Orren A, Kipps A, Dowdle EB, Shearing S and Falls E (1979) Serum complement concentrations, nutritional status and the outcome of Measles and Measles Pneumonia. S Afr Med J 55, 538–543

Osuntokun BO (1975) The traditional basis of neuropsychiatric practice among the Yorubas of Nigeria. Trop Geogr Med 27, 422–430

Palade GE (1952) A study of fixation for electronmicroscopy. J Exp Med 95, 285–298

Papp K (1954) Contagion des virus à travers une conjonctive intacte. Rougeole, oreillons, rubéole. Rev d'Imm Ther Antimicr 18, 380–390

Papp K (1956) Expériences prouvant que la voie d'infection de la rougeole est la contamination de la muqueuse conjonctivale. Rev d'Imm Thér Antimicr 20, 27–36

Papp C (1957) Voie d'infection du virus de la rougeole. Arch Fr Pédiat 14, 1049–1052

Passmore JW and King JH (1955) Vital staining of conjunctiva and cornea. Review of literature and critical study of certain dyes. Arch Ophthal 53, 568–574

Patwardhan VN (1969) Hypovitaminosis A and epidemiology of xerophthalmia. Amer J Clin Nutr 22, 1106–1118

Petzetakis M (1950) Les troubles oculaires pendant la trophopénie. La kératite superficielle trophopénique (kératopathie épithéliale). Presse Méd 58, 1082–1084

Pfister RR and Renner ME (1978) The corneal and conjunctival surface in vitamin A deficiency: a scanning electron microscope study. Invest Ophthal 17, 874–883

Phillips CM (1961) Blindness in Africans in Northern Rhodesia. Central Afr J Med 7, 153–158

Pillat A (1931) Über eine eigenartige Pigmentierung der Bindehaut bei den verschiedenen Formen der Vitamin A-Mangelerkrankung der Erwachsenen. Graefes Arch Ophthal 127, 575–597

Pillat A (1933) Production of pigment in the conjunctiva in night blindness, prexerosis, xerosis and keratomalacia of adults. Arch Ophthal 9, 25–47

Pirie A (1976) Xerophthalmia. Invest Ophthal 15, 417–422

Pirie A (1978) Effect of Vitamin A on the cornea. Trans Ophthal Soc UK 98, 357–360

Pirie A, Werb Z and Burleigh MC (1975) Collagenase and other proteinases in the cornea of the retinol-deficient rat. Brit J Nutr 34, 297–310

Poskitt EME (1971) Effect of measles on plasma-albumin levels in Ugandan village children. Lancet II, 68–70

Prause JU (1976) Collagenolysis of rat tail tendons by crude corneal collagenase and clostridiopeptidase A. Graefes Arch Ophthal 199, 249–254

Quéré MA (1964) Les complications oculaires de la rougeole, cause majeure de cécité chez l'enfant en pays tropical. Ophthalmologica 148, 107–120

Quéré MA, Satgé P, Graveline J, Charnay C, Diallo J and Blatt C (1967) Les kératopathies infantiles dans les Kwashiorkors et les dénutritions graves en Afrique tropicale. Bull Soc Fr Ophtal 80, 68–77

Rácz J (1965) Fälle von Koma-Keratitis. Graefes Arch Ophthal 168, 90–96

Rahi AHS and Garner A (1976) Immunopathology of the eye. Blackwell Scientific Publications, Oxford, London, Edinburgh, Melbourne

Rao KV and Singh D (1970) An evaluation of the relationship between nutritional status and anthropometric measurements. Amer J Clin Nutr 23, 83–93

Reddy V, Mohanram M and Raghuramulu N (1979) Serum Retinol-Binding-Protein and Vitamin A levels in malnourished children. Acta Paediatr Scan 68, 65–69

Reddy V and Srikantia SG (1966) Serum vitamin A in Kwashiorkor. Amer J Clin Nutr 18, 105–109

Regensburg NI and Henkes HE (1976) Measles (morbilli) and ocular complications. Docum Ophthal 40, 287–300

Rentier B, Hooghe-Peters EL and Dubois-Dalcq M (1978) Electron microscopic study of measles virus infection: cell fusion and hemadsorption. J. Virology 28, 567–577

Robbins FC (1962) Measles: Clinical features. Amer J Dis Child 103, 96–102

Roberts GBS and Bain AD (1958) The pathology of measles. J Path Bact 76, 111–118

Rodger FC (1959) Blindness in West Africa. London, Lewis and Co

Rodger FC, Dhir PK and Hosain ATMM (1960) Night blindness in the tropics. Arch Ophthal 63, 927–935

Rodger FC, Saiduzzafar H, Grover AD and Fazal A (1964) Nutritional lesions of the external eye and their relationship to plasma levels of vitamin A and the light thresholds. Acta Ophthal 42, 1–24

Rodrigues MR, Lennette DA, Arentsen JJ and Thompson C (1979) Methods for rapid detection of human ocular viral infections. Ophthalmology 86, 452–464

Roels OA, Trout M and Guha A (1965) The effect of vitamin A deficiency and dietary α-tocopherol on the stability of rat-liver lysosomes. Biochem J 97, 353–359

Rosen E (1949) The importance of the cornea in virus diseases. Ophthalmologica 118, 81–101

Rowsey JJ, Nisbet RM, Swedo JL and Katona L (1976) Corneal collagenolytic activity in rabbit polymorphonuclear leukocytes. J. Ultrastruct Res 57, 10–21

Roy FH (1974) Xerophthalmia. J Pediat Ophthal 11, 84–85

Ruckle G and Rogers KD (1957) Studies with measles virus. II. Isolation of virus and systems. Immunology 78, 330–340

Ruckle G and Rogers KD (1957) Studies with measles virus. II. Isolation of virus and immunologic studies in persons who have had the natural disease. J Immunol 78, 341–355

Sandford-Smith JH and Whittle HC (1979) Corneal ulceration following measles in Nigerian children. Brit J Ophthal 63, 720–724

Sauter JJM (1976) Xerophthalmia and measles in Kenya. Thesis. Groningen, van Denderen

Schappert-Kimmijser J (1959) De blindheidsoorzaken in Nederland. Publicatie van de Gezondheidsorganisatie TNO. Assen, Van Gorcum

Scheffel PD (1964) Ophthalmologie im Südafrikanischen Busch. Klin Mbl Augenheilk 144, 286–292

Scheifele DW and Forbes CE (1972) Prolonged giant cell excretion in severe African measles. Pediatrics 50, 867–873

Scheifele DW and Forbes CE (1973) The biology of measles in African children. East Afr Med J 50, 169–173

Schoental R (1972) Prevention or cure? Use of toxic herbs and geographic pathology. Trop Geogr Med 24, 194–198

Schwandt P, Fateh-Moghadam A, Richter W and Sandel P (1979) Retinol Binding Protein in malnutrition. The Lancet II, 794

Scrimshaw NS, Taylor CE and Gordon JE (1959) Interactions of nutrition and infection. Amer J Med Sci 237, 367–403

Sellmeyer E, Bhettay E, Truswell AS, Meyers OL and Hansen JDL (1972) Lymphocyte transformation in malnourished children. Arch Dis Childh 47, 429–435

Sergiev PG, Ryazantseva NE and Shroit IG (1960) The dynamics of pathological processes in experimental measles in monkeys. Acta Virol 4, 265–273

Shah U, Banerji KL, Nanavati AND and Mehta NA (1972) A test survey of measles in a rural community in India. Bull WHO 46, 130–138

Shapland CD (1946) Ocular disturbances associated with malnutrition. J Royal Army Med Corps 87, 253–265

Sheikh ME (1960) Vitamin deficiencies in relation to the eye. Brit J Ophthal 44, 406–414

Sherman FE and Ruckle G (1958) In vivo and in vitro cellular changes specific for measles. Arch Pathol 65, 587–599

Shetty PS, Jung RT, Watrasiewicz KE and James WPT (1979) Rapid-turnover transport proteins: an index of subclinical protein-energy malnutrition. The Lancet II, 230–232

Silverstein AM (1974) The immunologic modulation of infectious disease pathogenesis. Invest Ophthal 13, 560–571

Sinabulya PM (1976) An assessment of the extent of blindness in Machakos district. East Afr Med J 2, 64–73

Sinha BN (1966) The influence of protein on keratomalacia. J Indian Med Ass 47, 55–63

Sinha DP (1977) Measles and malnutrition in a West Bengal village. Trop Geogr Med 29, 125–134

Slansky HH, Gnädinger MC, Itoi M and Dohlman CH (1969) Collagenase in corneal ulcerations. Arch Ophthal 82, 108–111

Smelser GK and Ozanics V (1945) Effect of local anesthetics on cell division and migration following thermal burns of cornea. Arch Ophthal 34, 271–277

Smith FR, Goodman DS, Zaklama MS, Gabr MK, Maraghy SE and Patwardhan VN (1973) Serum vitamin A, retinol-binding protein, and prealbumin concentrations in protein-calorie malnutrition. I. A functional defect in hepatic retinol release. Amer J Clin Nutrit 26, 973–981

Smith FR, Goodman DS, Arroyave G and Viteri F (1973) Serum vitamin A, retinol-binding protein, and prealbumin concentrations in protein-calorie malnutrition. II. Treatment including supplemental vitamin A. Amer J Clin Nutr 26, 982–987

Smith FR, Suskind R, Thanangkul O, Leitzmann C, Goodman DS and Olson RE (1975) Plasma vitamin A, retinol-binding protein and prealbumin concentrations in protein-calorie malnutrition. III. Response to varying dietary treatments. Amer J Clin Nutr 28, 732–738

Smythe PM, Brereton-Stiles GG, Grace HJ, Mafoyane A, Schonland M, Coovadia HM, Loening WEK, Parent MA and Vos GH (1971) Thymolymphatic deficiency and depression of cell-mediated immunity in protein-calorie malnutrition. Lancet II, 939–943

Somerset EJ and Ghose N (1951) Blindness in India. Proc All India Ophthal Soc 12, 265–311

Sommer A (1975) Epidemiology in the design and evaluation of blindness control programs. Trans Amer Acad Ophthal Otolaryng 79, 447–452

Sommer A, Faich G and Quesada J (1975) Mass distribution of vitamin A and the prevention of keratomalacia. Amer J Ophthal 80, 1073–1080

Sommer A, Quesada J, Doty M and Faich G (1975) Xerophthalmia and anterior-segment blindness among preschool-age children in El Salvador. Amer J Ophthal 80, 1066–1072

Sommer A, Toureau S, Cornet P, Midy C and Pettiss ST (1976) Xerophthalmia and anterior segment blindness. Amer J Ophthal 82, 439–446

Sommer A (1978) Field guide to the detection and control of xerophthalmia. Geneva, World Health Organization

Sommer A (1980) Conjunctival xerosis. Letter to the editor. Am J Clin Nutr 33, 1313–1314

Sommer A, Tjakrasudjatma S, Djunaedi E and Green WR (1978) Vitamin A-responsive panocular xerophthalmia in a healthy adult. Arch Ophthal 96, 1630–1634

Sprunt DH and Flanigan CC (1956) The effect of malnutrition on the susceptibility of the host to viral infection. J Exp Med 104, 687–706

Spyratos Sp (1949) Héméralopie et altérations oculaires par carence en Grèce pendant les années 1941–1945. Ann d'Oculist 182, 672–685

Srikantia SG and Reddy V (1970) Effect of a single massive dose of vitamin A on serum and liver levels of the vitamin. Amer J Clin Nutr 23, 114–118

Srivastava SP and Nema HV (1963) Optic neuritis in measles. Brit J Ophthal 47, 180–181

Starr S and Berkovich S (1964) Effects of measles, gamma-globulin-modified measles and vaccine measles on the tuberculin test. New Engl J Med 270, 386–391

Stock EL and Aronson SB (1970) Corneal immune globulin distribution. Arch Ophthal 84, 355–359

Sullivan WR, McCulley JP and Dohlman CH (1973) Return of goblet cells after vitamin A therapy in xerosis of the conjunctiva. Amer J Ophthal 75, 720–725

Suringa WR, Bank LJ and Ackerman AB (1970) Role of measles virus in skin lesions and Koplik's spots. New Engl J Med 283, 1139–1142

Swiet M de, Fayers P and Cooper L (1977) Effect of feeding habit on weight in infancy, Lancet I, 892–894

Tajima M and Kudow S (1976) Morphology of the Warthin-Finkeldey giant cells in monkeys with experimentally induced measles. Acta Path Jap 26, 367–380

Taylor JE, Johnson DS and Dorsey WR (1966) The effect of live measles virus vaccine given with immune human globulin on measles keratitis. J Pediat Ophthal 3, 35–37

Thoft RA (1978) Role of the ocular surface in destructive corneal disease. Trans Ophthal Soc UK 98, 339–342

Thygeson P (1947) Marginal corneal infiltrates and ulcers. Trans Amer Acad Ophthal Otolaryng 52, 198–209

Thygeson P (1947) Clinical signs of diagnostic importance in conjunctivitis. J Amer Med Ass 133, 437–441

Thygeson P (1950) Superficial punctate keratitis. JAMA 144, 1544–1549

Thygeson P (1957) Present status of the viral keratoconjunctivitis problem. Amer J Ophthal 43, 3–10

Thygeson P (1959) Ocular viral diseases. Med Clin N Amer 43, 1419–1440

Thygeson P (1961) Further observations on superficial punctate keratitis. Arch Ophthal 66, 158–162

Tompkins V and Macauley JC (1955) A characteristic cell in nasal secretions during prodromal measle. J Amer Med Ass 157, 711

Trantas (1900) Complications oculaires rares de la rougeole. Ann d'Oculist 123, 390

Trantas (1903) Sur la kératite examthématique ponctuée superficielle pendant la rougeole. Ann d'Oculist 130, 97–112

Vahlquist A, Peterson PA and Wibell L (1973) Metabolism of the vitamin A transporting protein complex. I. Turnover studies in normal persons and in patients with chronic renal failure. Europ J Clin Invest 3, 352–362

Vahlquist A, Rask L, Peterson PA and Berg F (1975) The concentrations of retinol-binding protein, prealbumin, and transferrin in the sera of newly delivered mothers and children of various ages. Scand J Clin Lab Invest 35, 569–575

Valenton MJ and Tan RV (1975) Secondary ocular bacterial infection in hypovitaminosis A xerophthalmia. Amer J Ophthal 80, 673–677

Vanley GT, Leopold IH and Gregg TH (1977) Interpretation of tear film breakup. Arch Ophthal 95, 445–448

Vasantha L (1969) Labile collagen content in the skin in Kwashiorkor. Clin Chim Acta 26, 277–280

Vaughan DG (1954) Xerophthalmia. Arch Ophthal 51, 789–798

Venkataswamy G (1967) Ocular manifestations of vitamin A deficiency. Brit J Ophthal 51, 854–859

Vijayaraghavan K, Sarma KVR, Reddy V and Bhaskaram P (1978) Rose bengal staining for detection of conjunctival xerosis in nutrition surveys. Amer J Clin Nutr 31, 892–894

Vogel LC, Muller AS, Odingo RS, Onyango Z and de Geus A (eds)(1974) Health and disease in Kenya. East African Literature Bureau, Nairobi, Dar es Salaam, Kampala

Voorhoeve AM, Muller AS, Schulpen TWJ, Gemert W, Valkenburg HA and Ensering HE (1977) Agents affecting health of mother and child in a rural area of Kenya. III. The epidemiology of measles. Trop Geogr Med 29, 429–440

Voorhoeve HWA (1966) Xerophthalmia in the presence of Kwashiorkor in Nigeria. Trop Geogr Med 18, 15–19

Waterlow JC (1972) Classification and definition of protein-calorie malnutrition. Brit med J 3, 566–569

Waterlow JC and Payne PR (1975) The protein gap. Nature 258, 113–117

Watson I (1976) Pulmonary complications of measles. Brit med J 2, 945

Weekers L (1955) Le rôle des virus endormis dans la pathogénie de certaines kératites. Arch d'Ophtal 15, 839–845

Weisz FH (1972) On delegation in medicine and dentistry, Samson Uitgeverij, Alphen a.d. Rijn- Brussel

Whitehead RG, Frood JDL and Poskitt EME (1971) Value of serum-albumin measurements in nutritional surveys. Lancet II, 287–289

Whitehead RG and Alleyne GAO (1972) Pathophysiological factors of importance in protein-calorie malnutrition. Brit med Bull 28, 72–78

Whitehead RG, Coward WA and Lunn PG (1973) Serum-albumin concentration and the onset of Kwashiorkor. Lancet I, 63—66

Whittle HC, Sandford-Smith S, Kogbe OI, Dossetor J and Duggan M (1979) Severe ulcerative herpes of mouth and eye following measles. Trans Royal Soc Trop Med Hyg 73, 66—69

WHO (1973) The Prevention of Blindness. WHO Technical Report Series no 518

WHO (1973) Prevention of Blindness. WHO Chronicle 27, 21—27

WHO (1976) Vitamin A Deficiency and Xerophthalmia. Technical Report Series no 590

WHO (1978) Prevention of Blindness. WHO Wkly Epidem Rec 23, 165—168

WHO (1979) Guidelines for programmes for the prevention of blindness

WHO (1979) Blindness Surveillance. WHO Wkly Epid Rec No 32—36

Williams CD (1933) A nutritional disease of childhood associated with a maize diet. Arch Dis Childh 8, 423—433

Williams CD, Oxon BM and Lond H (1935) Kwashiorkor. A nutritional disease of children associated with a maize diet. Lancet II, 1151—1152

Wilson D, Bressani R and Scrimshaw NS (1961) Infection and nutritional status. I. The effect of chickenpox on nitrogen metabolism in children. Amer J Clin Nutr 9, 154—163

Wilson JR and Dubois RO (1923) Report of a fatal case of keratomalacia in an infant, with postmortem examination. Amer J Dis Child 26, 431—446

Wilson WS, Duncan AJ and Jay JL (1975) Effect of benzalkonium chloride on the stability of the precorneal tear film in rabbit and man. Brit J Ophthal 59, 667—669

Wilterdink JB (Ed)(1979) Medische Virologie. Bohn, Scheltema en Holkema, Utrecht

Witmer R and Moser R (1951) Sympathische Ophthalmie (s.O.) und Masern. Ophthalmologica 121, 175—176

Wolbach SB and Howe PR (1933) Epithelial repair in recovery from vitamin A deficiency. J Exp Med 57, 511—529

Yamagami I.(1971) Electron-microscopic study on the cornea. II. Electron-microscopic observation of arthus phenomenon in the cornea. Jap J Ophthal 15, 192—203

Yap-Kie-Tiong (1956) Protein deficiency in keratomalacia. Brit J Ophthal 40, 502—503

Yudkin AM and Lambert RA (1923) Pathogenesis of the ocular lesions produced by a deficiency of vitamine A. J Exp Med 38, 17—28

Summary

Introduction

In many developing countries measles is a very serious disease with a considerable morbidity and a high mortality (5 à 10%). An important complication is "Post-Measles-Blindness" which occurs in around 1% of the children affected with measles.

Protein Energy Malnutrition and/or Vitamin A Deficiency are commonly held responsible for this Post-Measles-Blindness. Also a bacterial superinfection is frequently mentioned. The significance of the routinely used traditional African ocular medicines is controversial.

None of the mentioned pathogenetic mechanisms explains why this corneal blindness occurs preferentially after measles and is only incidentally mentioned in connection with other diseases of childhood like malaria, meningitis, whooping cough, chickenpox or tuberculosis.

No good explanation for the epidemiological association between measles and corneal blindness is available, but it could only be self-evident to suppose that measles itself might do something directly to the cornea. This might initiate a chain of events, ultimately leading to corneal blindness. "Ophthalmology has neglected measles" (Quéré 1964) and it is the purpose of this study to fill this gap partially. Hopefully the results will be useful for the prevention of Post-Measles-Blindness.

Methods

The most important part of this investigation is the longitudinal study as to the involvement of the cornea in early measles. This work was done in a 150 bed Mission Hospital during a measles epidemic in the second half of 1976. 148 Children, admitted to the isolation ward, under the clinical diagnosis of measles — in many cases the diagnosis was confirmed by a positive anti-measles IgM in the serum — were daily examined with a hand held slitlamp-microscope. Further ophthalmological examinations were unfeasible in these mostly severely ill children.

For the demonstration of epithelial lesions in the conjunctiva and cornea the vital stains Rose Bengal, Lissamine Green and fluorescein were used. Rose Bengal and Lissamine Green stain damaged and degenerated cells, whereas fluorescein stains intercellular spaces, accessible to the dye in case of a damaged epithelium. Conjunctival biopsies and some corneae were sent to The Netherlands for pathological examination and immunofluorescence tests.

Ocular signs of measles

The conjunctiva is involved in the measles in two ways: first, in the prodromal fase virus multiplication takes place in the subepithelial lymphoid tissue, resulting in the characteristic conjunctivits, and second, more or less concomitant with the rash characteristic ,strictly epithelial lesions appear in the exposed parts of the bulbar conjunctiva. The size of these lesions is 0.2–0.4 mm and they have a limited lifespan of only some days. They can only be made visible with the use of vital stains.

These lesions appear to cross over the limbus to occupy the cornea, at first the periphery, later on the corneal centre. In the meantime the conjunctival lesions have healed. The last corneal lesions were observed 11 days after the outbreak of the rash. This measles-keratitis has, because of its strictly epithelial character, no permanent sequelae.

This measles-keratitis was observed in 76% of the 148 children. In 4% of the children with keratitis, the smaller lesions merge into larger macro-erosions, which also heal without permanent sequelae with appropriate treatment.

In some other children – mainly very severely ill – exposure ulcers were observed. Exposure is also a factor in the pathogenesis of some of the earlier mentioned macro-erosions.

The clinical picture of the measles-keratitis suggests, that it is caused by the measles virus. Immunofluorescent tests and electronmicroscopical examination of 10 conjunctival biopsies and 1 cornea demonstrated the presence of measles virus in the epithelium and keratocytes of the corneal stroma.

Measles-keratitis and nutritional status

Complications of measles are generally ascribed to Protein Energy Malnutrition, but the possibility exists that also *signs* of a disease are in their extent and/or severity dependent on the nutritional status. To test this last possibility also in the case of measles-keratitis a quantitative scoring system for the measles-keratitis was devised. The outcome was compared with anthropometric and biochemical parameters of the nutritional status. In our material no association could be demonstrated between the extent of the measles-keratitis and the nutritional status of the affected children. This finding is one reason more to suppose that the occurrence of the measles-keratitis will not be limited to children in developing countries: probably measles-keratitis is a sign of measles in the majority of *all* children with measles.

The pathogenesis of Post-Measles-Blindness

Post-Measles-Blindness is in my opinion caused by a cooperation of three factors: measles, malnutrition and treatment. In this study we demonstrated that at least 76% of all children with measles have a measles-keratitis, in 4% of them leading to a corneal macro-erosion. To the keratitis are added the problems of exposure. This makes the cornea more open to secundary infection and further complications.

In this respect it is remarkable, that in the corneal stroma of an eye, lost due to panophthalmitis after measles, on electronmicroscopical examination particles were found, resembling viral strands. The significance of this isolated finding is at this moment unclear.

An acute Protein Energy Malnutrition (= kwashiorkor) is frequently caused by measles. This causes an extreme biochemical disturbance, resulting in an impaired immunological defence system and a diminished protein synthesis. This last factor might cause a destabilisation of the corneal collagen. The cornea is in danger by both mechanisms.

The significance of traditional African ocular medicines is controversial. The opinions in this respect vary from "nonsense" to the "most important cause" of Post-Measles-Blindness. I am personally convinced that in some cases they add an important factor to an already endangered cornea.

It was also demonstrated, that the frequent application of tetracycline prevents the development of early corneal complications.

In my opinion the measles-keratitis is the explanation for the existence of Post-Measles-Blindness, whereas the epidemiology of malnutrition explains why it occurs in underpriviliged populations.

Prevention

The prevention of Post-Measles-Blindness must take all these factors into account: a combined attack by measlesvaccination, topical protection of the cornea and improvement of the nutritional status will eventually eradicate Post-Measles-Blindness.

Samenvatting

Inleiding

In menig ontwikkelingsland is mazelen nog steeds een ernstige kinderziekte. Samen met andere infectieziekten, zoals malaria, menigitis, kinkhoest, gastro-enteritis en tuberculose, is het een belangrijke oorzaak voor de hoge kindersterfte. Vrijwel altijd speelt daarbij ondervoeding (Protein-Energy-Malnutrition) een belangrijke rol.

Ook blindheid op de kinderleeftijd is in veel ontwikkelings-landen een aanzienlijk probleem. Bij de niet-aangeboren blindheid is deze veelal corneaal gelokaliseerd en het is opmerkelijk, dat in een groot percentage der gevallen een verband met mazelen wordt aangegeven; de andere kinderziekten worden steeds incidenteel als veroorzaker van blindheid vermeld.

Als uiteindelijke oorzaak van deze corneale blindheid na mazelen wordt veelal een Vitamine A deficientie beschouwd. Een bacteriële superinfectie is een andere vaak genoemde oorzaak. De rol van potentieel toxische Afrikaanse geneesmiddelen is evenwel meer omstreden.

Een goede verklaring voor het epidemiologische verband tussen mazelen en corneale blindheid ontbreekt. De gebruikelijke verklaring is, dat door de mazeleninfectie bij een te voren latent ondervoed kind een Vitamine A gebrek manifest wordt; mazelen is dan de aanleiding tot een Vitamine A afhankelijke keratomalacie.

Hiermee is nog niet verklaard waarom dit juist bij mazelen zou gebeuren. Het zou daarom voor de hand liggen te veronderstellen, dat mazelen zelf een direct effect heeft op de cornea, wat dan een eerste fase zou kunnen zijn van een tot blindheid leidende corneale complicatie. Onder- en/of wanvoeding spelen daarbij waarschijnlijk een belangrijke rol. In deze studie kan slechts een klein facet van de onderlinge samenhang tussen mazelen en voedingstoestand ter sprake komen.

Methodiek

Dit proefschrift is het verslag van een longitudinaal onderzoek naar de betrokkenheid van de cornea bij mazelen. Het belangrijkste deel van het onderzoek werd in de tweede helft van 1976 verricht in een 150 beds Missie ziekenhuis in West-Kenya. Tijdens de toen heersende mazelen-epidemie werden 148 kinderen opgenomen op de isolatie-afdeling. De diagnose mazelen werd op klinische gronden gesteld en bij een groot aantal van hen bevestigd door een positieve test op anti-mazelen IgM in het serum.

Deze 148 kinderen werden dagelijks met de handspleetlamp bekeken. Een uitgebreider oogheelkundig onderzoek was bij deze ernstig zieke kinderen niet doenlijk.

Om laesies in het epitheel van conjunctiva en cornea aan te tonen werd gebruik gemaakt van de vitale kleurstoffen Bengaals Rood (later Lissamine Groen) en fluoresceine. De eerste kleuren beschadigde epitheelcellen, fluoresceine daarentegen diffundeert in de intercellulaire ruimten bij een aanwezig epitheel defect.

Oogheelkundige symptomen van mazelen

De conjunctiva bleek op twee verschillende manieren mee te doen met de mazelen:

(a) Tijdens de prodromale fase heeft een subepitheliale virusvermenigvuldiging plaats, in de lymfoide laag van de conjunctiva, wat de oorzaak is van de voor de prodromale mazelen kenmerkende conjunctivitis.

(b) Min of meer samenvallend met het uitbreken van de mazelen rash, traden kenmerkende laesies van het epitheel op, veelal zonder dat zich daar ter plaatse ontstekingsverschijnselen als vaatverwijding voordeden.

De conjunctivale epitheliale laesies waren gelokaliseerd in de lidspleet, waren 0,2 à 0,4 mm groot en hadden een kenmerkende vorm. Hun levensduur was slechts enkele dagen. Deze laesies waren alleen zichtbaar te maken door het gebruik van vitale kleurstoffen.

In de volgende dagen verplaatsten deze laesies zich over de limbus naar de cornea, waarbij veelal het centrum van de cornea het laatst was aangedaan.

12 Dagen na het uitbreken van de rash werden geen corneale laesies meer aangetroffen. De conjunctivale epitheliale laesies waren al eerder verdwenen. Deze mazelen-keratitis liet, vanwege zijn strikt epitheliale verloop, geen corneale littekens achter.

Deze mazelen-keratitis werd gezien bij 76% van de 148 kinderen. Bij 4% van de kinderen met keratitis conflueerden de kleine laesies tot grotere macro-ersosies. Ook deze erosies genazen zonder corneale littekens met de gebruikelijke conservatieve behandeling.

Alles duidde erop dat de mazelen-keratitis een virale keratitis was. Dit kon door laboratorium onderzoek worden bevestigd. In conjunctiva biopten kon door middel van immunofluorescentie mazelen antigeen worden aangetoond in het conjunctiva epitheel. In conjunctiva biopten, bewerkt voor de electronen microscoop, werd subepitheliaal virus aangetroffen in lymfocyten. De ontwikkeling van de gewone mazelen keratitis tot een macro-erosie kon, zowel bij pathologisch anatomisch als electronen microscopisch onderzoek van conjunctiva biopsen en een mazelen cornea, aannemelijk worden gemaakt door het aantonen van sterk verminderde cellulaire adhaesie.

Dit alles leidde tot de conclusie, dat een subepitheliale conjunctivitis en een epitheliale conjunctivo-keratitis beschouwd dienen te worden als symptomen van mazelen.

Mazelen-keratitis en voedingstoestand

Symptomen van mazelen zijn in hun ernst en omvang, evenals de complicaties, gecorreleerd met de voedingstoestand van de mazelen patientjes. Om deze mogelijke correlatie voor de mazelen-keratitis (als *symptoom* van mazelen) na te gaan, werd een quantitatief scoringssysteem voor de keratitis ontworpen. Deze scores werden vergeleken met enkele biochemische en anthropometrische parameters voor de voedingstoestand. Er kon evenwel in ons materiaal geen verband worden vastgesteld tussen de omvang van de mazelen-keratitis en de voedingstoestand.

De pathogenese van blindheid na mazelen

Blindheid na mazelen wordt veroorzaakt door een interactie van de 3 factoren: mazelen, ondervoeding en behandeling.

a. *Mazelen.* In deze studie konden we aantonen dat tenminste 76% van de kinderen een mazelen-keratitis doormaakte, terwijl 4% van alle kinderen een verdergaande beschadiging van de cornea (hetzij een erosie, hetzij een uitdrogings-ulcus) vertoonde. Alleen al hierdoor is de cornea ontvankelijker voor het optreden van secundaire infecties en verdere complicaties. Bij electronen-microscopisch onderzoek van een cornea, afkomstig van een oog, verloren na mazelen, werden in de keratocyten partikels aangetroffen, welke mogelijk virus-partikels zouden kunnen zijn. Deze bevinding was totaal onverwacht en op dit moment is de betekenis nog onduidelijk.

b. *Ondervoeding.* Bij het ontstaan van blindheid na mazelen speelt ondervoeding een zeer belangrijke rol. Een acute ondervoeding (kwashiorkor) kan geprovoceerd worden door mazelen. Deze geeft een extreme verstoring van biochemische processen, wat o.a. aanleiding kan zijn tot verminderde immunologische afweer en een destabilisering van collageen, wat op zijn beurt ook de cornea weer kwetsbaarder maakt.

c. *Lokale behandeling van de cornea.* Er zijn argumenten om aan te nemen, dat sommige inheemse Afrikaanse geneesmiddelen een schadelijk effect op de cornea zouden kunnen hebben. Sommigen vinden dit een onbelangrijke factor, terwijl anderen met stelligheid beweren dat het de belangrijkste oorzaak is van blindheid na mazelen. Ik ben er van overtuigd, dat sommige van deze geneesmiddelen een belangrijke schadelijke factor extra zijn.

Indien kinderen met mazelen echter consequent een oogzalf met een antibioticum kregen toegediend, traden aanmerkelijk minder complicaties op: zalf beschermde de cornea.

Preventie van blindheid na mazelen

Alle bovengenoemde factoren lenen zich als aangrijpingspunt voor de voorkoming van blindheid na mazelen: mazelenvaccinatie, verbetering van de voedingstoestand, het vermijden van sommige schadelijke handelwijzen en de bescherming van de cornea met zalf, zullen een drastische vermindering van de blindheid na mazelen te zien geven.

Résumé

Introduction

A l'opposé de la situation observeé en Europe et aux Etats-Unis la rougeole a des conséquences beaucoup plus graves dans les pays du Tiers-monde. Les symptômes sont souvent beaucoup plus graves et les complications sont plus fréquentes et la mortalité est élevée (5 à10%). La raison, pour laquelle je me suis attaché à ces recherches, est la prévention de la cécité cornéenne consécutive à la rougeole qui se produit environ chez 1% des enfants atteints.

On attribue la plupart du temps à l'origine de cette cécité cornéenne une sous-alimentation et un manque de vitamine A; on accorde aussi souvent comme cause une surinfection bactérielle. Le rôle, joué par des médicaments indigènes, à usage fréquent, est très discutable.

Cependant, il est à remarquer que cette forme de cécité se déclare après une rougeole alors qu'un rapport de cause à effet est rarement signalé dans les maladies telles que malaria, méningite, coqueluche, variole ou tuberculose dans les pays, couvrant le Tiers-monde. Il manque à cette relation épidémique une interprétation valable.

On pourrait être tenté d'établir que la rougeole a un effet, direct sur la cornée et déclenche une série de réactions consécutives lesquelles pourraient finalement amener à la cécité. Jusqu'à présent, on a fait très peu de recherches dans le sens de relation directe entre la rougeole et ses complications sur la cornée.

Le but de ces examens longitudinaux est une clarification d'idées à propos des effets de la rougeole sur la cornée, dans l'espoir que ces données pourront contribuer ainsi à la prévention de la cécité après la rougeole.

Méthode

La partie la plus importante de nos recherches – c'est à dire, une étude longitudinale consacrée à la relation de la cornée dans la phase aiguïe de la rougeole – fut faite dans un hôpital missionaire de 150 lits au Kenya-Ouest, pendant la seconde moitié de l'année 1976.

Pendant l'épidémie de rougeole, 148 enfants furent hospitalisés et mis en quarantaine. Le diagnostic de la rougeole a été établi par des symptômes cliniques et pour un grand nombre de ces cas, confirmés par un test positif à l'aide d'un IgM antirougeole dans le sang. On a observé quotidiennement ces 148 enfants grâce à une lampe à fente à main.

Il se révéla impossible de faire chez ces enfants gravement atteints un examen oculaire plus conséquent. Pour donner la preuve des lésions dans l'épithélium conjonctival et cornéen, on a fait l'emploi de colorants vitaux, Rose Bengal, plus tard Lissamine Verte et de fluoresceïne.

Les premiers teintent les cellules épithéliales lésées à l'opposé de la flouroesceïne qui se diffuse dans les espaces intercellulaires en présence d'un épithélium déficient.

Les symptômes oculaires de la rougeole

Il est apparu pendant ces recherches que la conjonctive était atteinte de deux façons différentes à compter avec un déroulement normal de la maladie; d'abord pendant la phase prodromale, il se crée une multiplication du virus dans le tissu lymfoïde de la conjonctive qui se manifeste cliniquement sous la forme d'une conjonctivite; en second lieu, simultanément à l'apparation du "rash" l'épithélium conjonctival laisse apparaître des lésions caractéristiques en l'absence de symptômes infectieux locaux, comme par exemple, une dilatation vasculaire.

Sur ce dernier symptôme va se centrer toute notre attention. Les lésions conjonctivales épithéliales nommées ici plus-haut, sont localisées dans la fente palpébrale; elles mesurent 0,2 à 0,4 mm. et elles ont une morphologie caractéristique avec une durée, limitée à quelques jours. On parvient à rendre ces lésions visibles grâce à l'emploi de colorants vitaux.

Ces lésions qui se déplacent les jours suivants vers la cornée, vont traverser de limbe pour se terminer à maintes reprises dans le centre de la cornée; 12 jours après l'éruption du "rash", on ne parvient pas à déceler des lésions cornéennes. Les lésions épithéliales de la conjonctive ont déjà effectué plus tôt leur disparation. Cette kératite dûe à la rougeole, du fait de la seule atteinte de l'épithélium, ne laisse pas de cicatrice sur la cornée.

On a pu observer la kératite dûe à la rougeole chez 76% des 148 enfants atteints. Les petites lésions confluent en macro-lésions chez 4% des enfants atteints de kératite.

Ces érosions guérissent sans cicatrice cornéenne grâce à un traitement habituel.

Chez quelques autres enfants pour la plupart gravement atteints, on va constater l'apparition d'un ulcère cornéen par dissiccation, résultant de la fermeture insuffisante des paupéres.

L'application routinière d'une pommade à tous les enfants atteints paraît être suffisante pour prévenir les érosions cornéennes aussi bien que les ulcères à base de dessication. Le tableau clinique de la kératite fait penser que ces lésions épithéliales dans la conjonctive et la cornée sont provoquées par le virus de la rougeole. On peut confirmer ces dires par un examen immuno-fluorescent et microscopique électronique de 10 biopsies conjonctivales et un examen microscopique électronique d'une cornée.

La kératite à rougeole et la nutrition

Une sous-alimentation est en général la cause des complications de la rougeole. Il est tout aussi possible que la gravité des symptômes de la rougeole est liée aux habitudes nutritives.

Pour affirmer cette possibilité pour la kératite à rougeole (comme symptôme de la rougeole), nous avons créé un système de score quantitatif ayant trait à la kératite, qui par après a été comparé avec des paramètres biochimiques et antropométriques de nutrition. On n'a pas pu établir une liaison entre la gravïté de kératite à rougeole et la nutrition.

Ce n'est pas pour cette seule raison, qu'on peut poser l'hypothèse que cette kératite chez les enfants atteints de rougeole, les frappe sans distinction d'habitat, dans les pays du Tiers-monde ou dans nos pays d'occident.

La genèse de la cécité après la rougeole

Ces données doivent contribuer à la conversion dans chaque théorie, au sujet de la genèse de la cécité cornéenne, bien que cela reste encore naturellement dans le domaine du spéculatif.

On peut démontrer dans cette étude qu'au moins 76% des enfants ont été atteints d'une kératite à rougeole, tandis que 4% de nombre total des enfants ont subi une détérioration de la cornée (soit qu'il s'agisse d'une érosion ou ulcère d'exposition).

Pour cette seule raison, la cornée est beaucoup plus sensibilisée aux infections secondaires et à d'autres complications. Au moyen d'une recherche microscopique-électronique d'une cornée, d'un œil perdu après une infection à rougeole, on a découvert des particules dans les kératocytes, lesquelles sont probablement des particules virales à rougeole.

Cette découverte est tout à fait inattendue et à l'heure qu'il est le sens en est encore confus. Le rôle principal, la rougeole mise à part, est joué par la malnutrition. Une sous-alimentation aigue (kwashiorkor) peut être provoquée par la rougeole.

Celle-ci mène à une perturbation grave des procès biochimiques qui peut conduire à une défense immunologique moindre de l'organisme et une perturbation du collagène, qui rend à son tour la cornée plus vulnérable.

Le sens qu'on veut accorder à l'emploi de médicaments ophtalmologiques africains et traditionnels, est cependent controversé. Certains ne prennent pas ce facteur en considération, alors que d'autres certifient que l'emploi de ceuxci est la cause primordiale de cécité, après une rougeole. Je suis tout à fait persuadé que ces médicaments y ajoutent souvent un facteur funeste.

Prévention

La cécité provoquée par la rougeole est probablement causée par une association de trois facteurs: la rougeole, la sous-alimentation et le traitement. La prévention devra se concentrer sur la vaccination contre la rougeole, la lutte contre la sous-alimentation et éviter l'usage de médicaments traditionnels funestes. Cela ne veut pas dire qu'il faut totalement en éliminer l'emploi.

La conclusion de cette thèse se résume sans peine: l'existence de la kératite à rougeole peut expliquer la cécité cornéenne de préference après une rougeole; l'épidémiologie de la sous-alimentation, la raison pour laquelle cela se produit seulement dans les pays du Tiers-monde.

Acknowledgements

This thesis would never have been completed if not a great number of institutions and persons had given their support and active cooperation. I owe them many thanks.

The Professor Weve Foundation (The Netherlands) with Prof. G.H.L. Zeegers and Dr. A.A.J.J. van der Eerden, made large contributions to the rural eye work in Western Kenya. They enabled me to work in Kenya for over three years and stimulated in every respect the continuation of this study.

The Dutch Ursuline Sisters (Bergen NH, The Netherlands) with Sisters Giovanni, Doreen and José, founded the Mukumu Mission Hospital and gave hospitality to the Professor Weve Foundation Eye Clinic. I have been the guest in their hospital.
I thank the doctors H.J.A. Lijftogt, H.R. Renkema, A.M. Renkema-de Boer and J.A. Hage for their stimulating support. Without the help of a great number of student nurses, the part on nutrition would never have been written.

The Medical Research Centre, Nairobi (Dpt. of the Royal Tropical Institute, Amsterdam) supported me with a vast amount of laboratory assistence. Miss H.L. Ensering did the virological, Miss M.M. van Rens the nutritional side of the work. Mr. W. Gemert took care of the statistical analysis, all under the stimulating interest of Dr. Th.A.C. Hanegraaf, director of the centre.

The Kenyan Government offered indispensable help. Dr. M.L. Odouri, Chief Paediatrician of the Kenyatta National Hospital, offered the possibility to examine his patients and to take biopsies. Dr. P. Muthiga, Paediatrician at the Kakamega Provincial Hospital, accepted, that the clinical trial was done in his measles-ward. The Director of Medical Services of the Ministry of Health, Dr. J.C. Likimani gave consent to perform the Shikusa Survey.

The P.W.F. Eye Clinic, with my friends Miss Passilidah Ongayo, Mr. John Gari, Mr. Bartholomew Nyakundi and Mr. Anthony Opondo supported me always and gave actual help where ever needed.

The Erasmus University (Dpt. of Pathology) Dr. F.J.W. ten Kate, Dr. V.D. Vuzevski and Prof. Dr. W.A. Manschot examined the conjunctival biopsies. Mrs. P. Delfos took care of the photographs. Dr. F.E. Nommensen of the dpt. of Virology made an indispensable contribution by the preparation and examination of conjunctival biopsies with immunofluorescence. Ir. P. Schmitz, dpt. of Medical Statistics offered valuable statistical help.

The Netherlands Ophthalmic Research Institute (Dpt. of Morphology) Drs. G.F.J.M. Vrensen and J.J.L. van der Want did an important work with the electronmicroscopy of conjunctival biopsies and corneas. Their contribution to this study is not easily overestimated.

The Rotterdam Eye Hospital where I did my residency under Prof. Dr. H.E. Henkes and Prof. Dr. A.Th.M. van Balen, supported me in every respect, when in Africa and later on back in Holland. The staff enabled me to finish the work. Agnes Wallaart (librarian) made a great contribution by compiling all of the literature and Mr. C.B. Schotel made the drawings.

Elly Berkers-Mecking, my secretary, typed and retyped the manuscript, with great accuracy.

Haaren, 18-2-1981

Legends to
COLOURPLATE I

Figure 3.3. The differential staining of Rose Bengal 1% and Fluorescein 1% in a case of herpetic keratitis. The Rose Bengal stains devitalized cells, whereas fluorescein is seen to diffuse into the surrounding epithelium. This herpetic keratitis was seen in a 4 years old Luhya girl, 4 weeks after the measles rash. She is – anthropometically – mildly malnourished, whereas the biochemical estimations are in the well-nourished range (Retinol Binding Protein 2.7, Albumin 3090). Traditional medicines had been applied (§ 4.4) (Pat P 172)

Figure 4.4.b. Descemetocele, with incarceration of the iris, in a 6 years old Elgeyo boy, two weeks after the outbreak of the measles rash. The child was well nourished, no nightblindness, no Bitot's spots. Traditional medicines had been applied. Pat Tamb VA 120

Figure 4.4.c. 2 years 8 months old, severely malnourished Luhya girl with a corneal perforation and secondary (?) infection, 2 weeks after the measles rash. The clinical impression "panophthalmitis" was confirmed on evisceration, when a purulent hyalitis was found. In the corneal stroma possibly measles virus could be detected on electron-microscopical examination (fig. 5.3.h). The serum albumin (2460 mg%) is rather low. The Retinol Binding Protein in the serum is normal (3.2) Pat Muk P 258

Figure 4.4.d. The same patient as fig. 4.4.c. Descemetocele, with incarceration of iris of the left eye, 2 weeks after the measles rash.

Figure 4.4.e. Hypopyonulcer in a malnourished Elgeyo boy, 16 months of age, 3 weeks after the outbreak of the rash. The hypopyon has an unusual localization: prior to examination the boy had been sleeping for several hours at his left hand side. The ulcer healed with conservative treatment. Traditional medicines had been applied. Pat Tamb P 273

Figure 4.4.f. Descemetocele in the right eye of a 8 years old girl, 4 weeks after a measles rash. This 8 years old Kalengin girl is overtly malnourished, and is treated for pulmonary tuberculosis. The left eye demonstrates a phlyctenular keratitis (fig. 4.4.g) Pat Tamb VA 28

Figure 4.4.g. The same patient as fig 4.4.f. The cornea of the left eye showed several phlyctenulae

Figure 4.4.h. Corneal perforation in a 7 months old Luo boy, 5 weeks after the measles rash. The child was breastfed. The Weight for Age is 77%. Pat SiaVA 16

Figure 4.4.i. Corneal staphyloma in an 18 months old, overfed girl, 2 months after the measles rash. Pat Bung VA 83

COLOURPLATE I

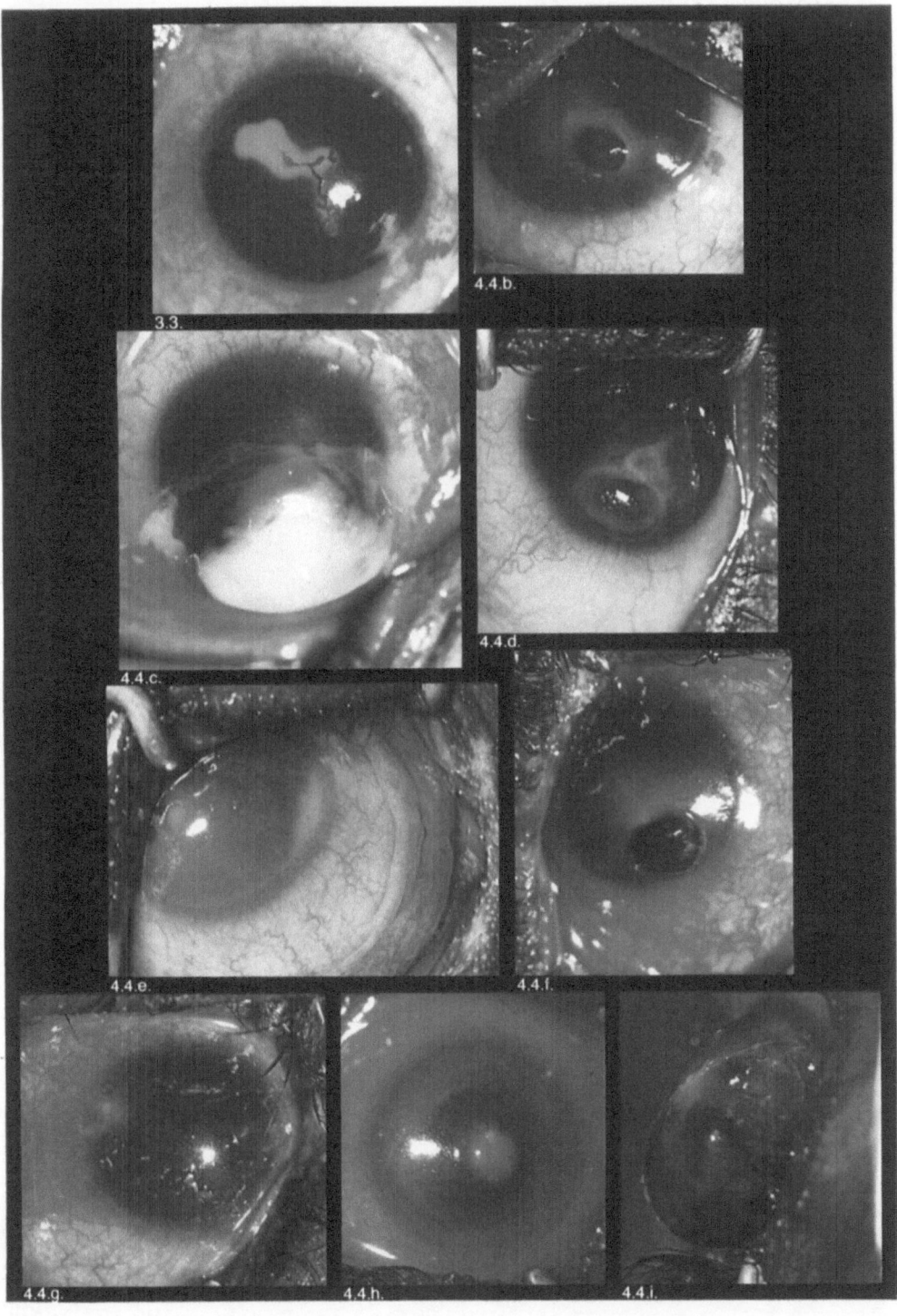

110

Legends to:
COLOURPLATE II *(see page 112)*

Figure 4.1.2.a. Conjunctival lesions intensely staining with Lissamine Green occurring in the early exanthematous stage of measles, localized in the interpalpebral fissure. (Pat M 234, day R + 1)

Figure 4.1.2.b. Larger magnification of the conjunctival epithelial lesions of early exanthematous measles, stained with Rose Bengal. Pat M 206, day R + 1

Figure 4.1.2.d. Conjunctival epithelial lesions are present in continuity with the same lesions in the cornea. It is difficult to show a good picture of this transition because of the extreme difference in contrast at the limbus. The conjunctival lesions are stained with Rose Bengal, the corneal lesions stain with fluorescein. Pat M 206, day R + 1

Figure 4.1.2.e. At this stage the measles keratitis is more or less restricted to the corneal perifery. Pat Cr 63, Day R + 2

Figure 4.1.2.f. The conjunctiva and limbus are now free. The keratitis is localized at the midperipheral and central parts of the cornea. Pat Cr 129, day R + 4

Figure 4.1.2.g. The last manifestation of the epithelial measles keratitis: only the centre of the cornea is involved. Pat M 18, day R + 3

Legends to:
COLOURPLATE III *(see page 113)*

Figure 4.2.1.a. Corneal erosion in a child with measles, 9 days after the outbreak of the rash, 3 days after the administration of 200.000 IU Vit. A. Pat K 19

Figure 4.2.1.b. Large central corneal erosion, surrounded by an extensive measles keratitis, 9 days after the outbreak of the rash. Pat M 149 (Electronmicroscopy in Fig 5.3.b and c)

Figure 4.2.2.a. (cfr Figure 4.2.2.b) Exposure ulcer in the cornea of a 4 years old boy, 3 weeks after outbreak of the rash. Pat M 117

Figure 5.1.2.b. Positive immunofluorescence test for measles antigen in the subepithelial tissue of a Lissamine Green negative biopsy. The yellow colour indicates the presence of measles antigen

Figure 5.1.2.c. The presence of measles virus antigen in the epithelium of a lissamine Green positive conjunctival biopsy is demonstrated by a positive immunofluorescence test

COLOURPLATE II

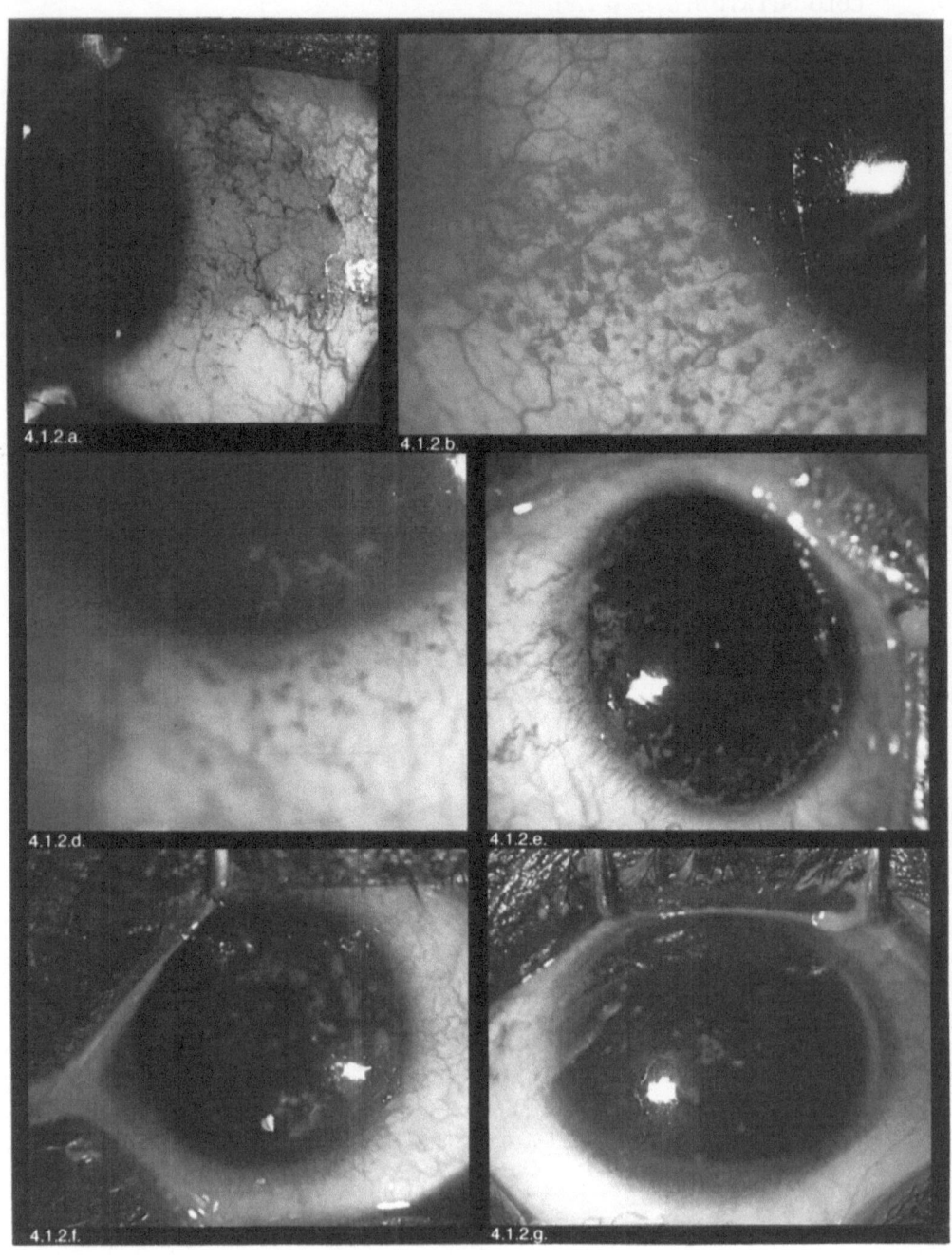

4.1.2.a.

4.1.2.b.

4.1.2.d.

4.1.2.e.

4.1.2.f.

4.1.2.g.

COLOURPLATE III

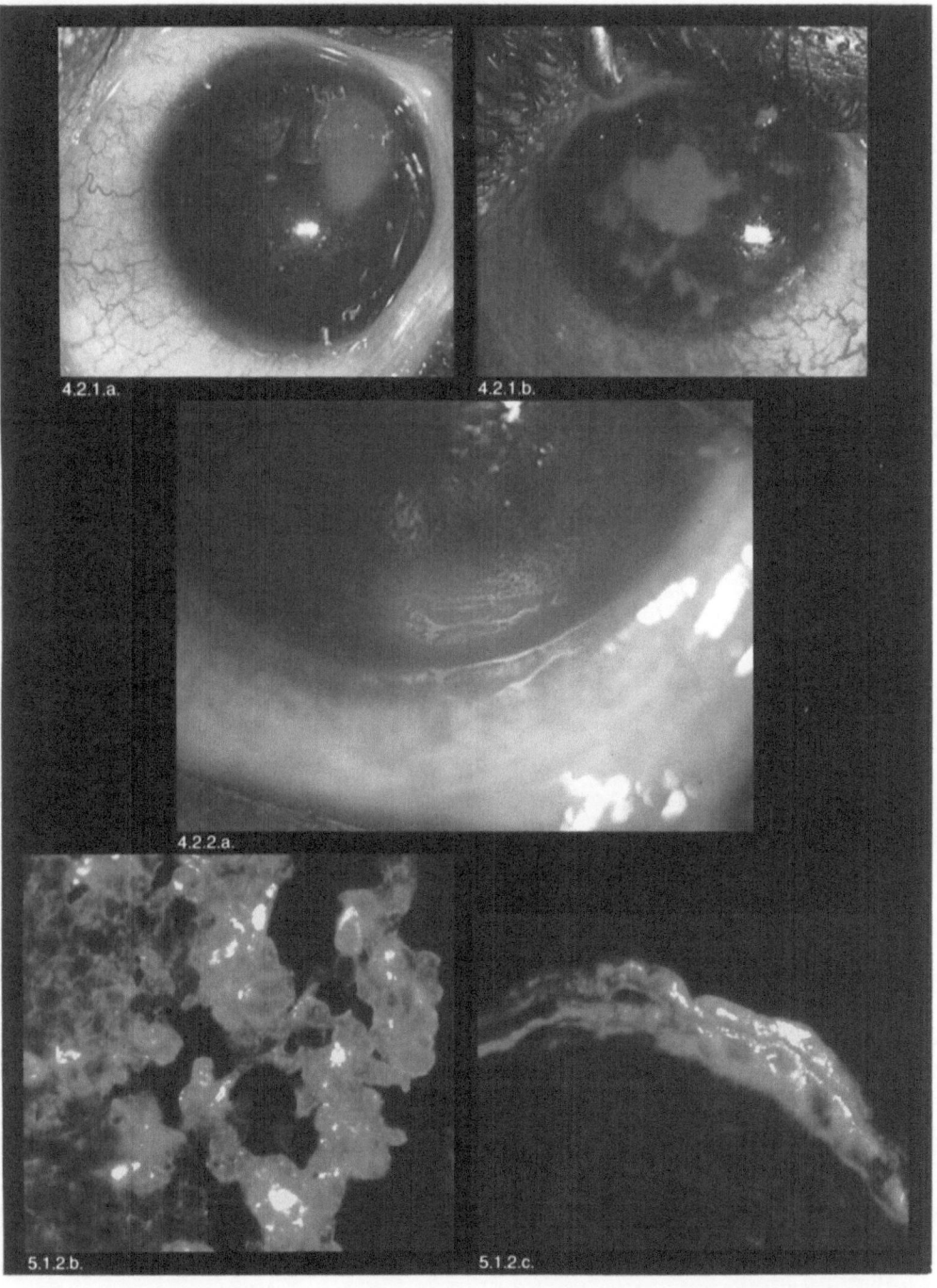

4.2.1.a.

4.2.1.b.

4.2.2.a.

5.1.2.b.

5.1.2.c.

APPENDIX

In this appendix the numerical data regarding the 148 patients in the group Mukumu I are tabulated. The methods used are described in §3.3 and 3.5.

The age is given in months.

H	=	height
H/A	=	height for age
W	=	weight
W/A	=	weight for age
W/H	=	weight for height
Vacc	=	history of vaccination against measles
Alb	=	Serum albumin. Normal value in European adults: 3,500–5,500 mg%.
RBP	=	Retinol Binding Protein. Normal value in European adults: 3–6 mg%.
Ker	=	Keratitis score
Adm	=	Data of admission compared to the day of outbreak of the rash (= R)
Obser	=	Observation period

For the calculation of H/A, W/A and W/H the Harvard standard as commonly in use in Kenya as the "Road to Health" is used.

Nr	Sex	Age	H	H/A	W	W/A	W/H	Vacc	Alb	RBP	Ker	Adm	Obser	Remarks
1	M	18						-	2625	2.9	2	R	7	
2	M	10			9.1	98		-	2850	2.0	0	3	9	
3	F	51	112	106	19.4	114	97	+	2550	2.2	-	1	2	
4	M	47	89	87	13.5	83	106	-	2870	1.4	9	2	8	
5	F	36							2430	1.3	0	3	6	
6	M	20	80	96	7.9	67	72	-			0	R	19	
7	M	48	96	93	10.5	63	72		<1500	<1.2	1	2	22	died, exposure ulcer
8	M	36							2985	1.9	7	3	18	
9	M	32						-	2070	2.2	2	4	6	
10	F	8			5.5	65			2348	1.8	4	4	16	
11	F	18							.3100	1.4	2	1	12	
12	F	14	66	86					2515	2.8	1	4	17	
13	M	11	67	91	7.5	78	94			1.9	6	3	13	
14	Non existent													
15	F	18						-	3390	1.8	8	1	6	
16	M	13	66	87	6.5	64	88	+	2205	2.2	1	-1	5	
17	M	21	81	96	8.5	71	75	-	2790	1.5	5	1	9	
18	M	48	Malnutrition					-	1300	1.3	16	1	6	died
19	F	28	82	91	8.7	66	77	-			9	4	8	
20	M	12	60	80	6.4	64	112	+	3450	1.4	7	3	12	
21	M	14							2065	2.0	0	1	5	
22	F	30	85	93					2820	2.4	5	4	5	
23	M	8	60	87	6.5	77	114	+	3310	2.1	6	2	14	
24	M	29	76	83	11.3	85	110	-	2820	1.3	0	3	7	
25	F	14	60	78	6.3	60	111	-	2120	1.3	4	R	8	
26	M	7	59	87	8.1	101	142	-	2895	1.7	4	4	8	
27	M	34	87	92	10.1	71	81	-	2840	2.7	0	1	6	
28	F	10	73	101	7.9	85	82	+			10	1	11	
29	F	29	88	96	10.8	81	86	-	2670	1.7	5	-1	7	
30	F	9	67	95	7.6	85	95	-	2095	<1.2	3	1	7	
31	F	17	72	89	8.7	79	94	-	2700	<1.2	0	1	6	
32	M	10	62	86	6.0	64	95	-	3065	2.5	8	1	14	
33	M	11	68	93	8.1	84	101	-	2640	1.3	0	2	13	
34	M	64	105	95	14.0	72	83	-	2755	2.5	5	R	9	
35	M	11	68	93	8.1	84	101	+	2045	<1.2	12	2	12	
36	F	108	129	97	20.3	70	77	-	2245	1.2	-	1	14	
37	F	67	104	91	15.3	74	92	-	3020	1.5	-	2	9	
38	F	9	66	93	6.7	75	91	+		1.2	+	1	9	died
39	F	48							2295	1.5	+	1	7	
40	F	55	105	98	15.3	87	91	-	2545	2.1	-	R	11	

Nr	Sex	Age	H	H/A	W	W/A	W/H	Vacc	Alb	RBP	Ker	Adm	Obser	Remarks
41	F	42	94	94	16.1	104	115	+	2060	<1.2	+	5	8	
42	Non existent													
43	F	19	80	97	10.0	87	91	-	2550	1.2	6	2	8	
44	F	34	78	82	8.3	61	78	-	1950	1.2	6	1	18	
45	F	19	84	102	9.9	86	83	-	3175	<1.2	12	7	7	
46	M	14	70	91	7.4	71	83	-	3085	1.7	18	1	11	
47	M	36	92	96	10.1	70	75		2070	1.2	-	3	1	died
48	M	14	70	91	8.1	78	91	-	2995	1.7	4	1	7	
49	M	36	90	94	11.6	80	90	+	2550	1.2	7	1	7	
50	M	23	74	86	9.0	74	94	-	2125	1.2	17	1	7	
51	M	72	99	84	15.5	71	101	-	2065	1.2	4	1	11	
52	F	8	62	90	4.9	58	78	-	2320	1.3	6	3	8	
53	F	49						-	3690	1.3	2	1	7	
54	F	28						-	3395	1.8	0	3	8	
55	M	12	76	102	9.1	91	89	-	3640	2.1	2	1	7	
56	F	138	140	95	25.0	66	78	-	2040	<1.2	5	2	7	
57	M	69			12.1	58		-	1815	<1.2	0	6	6	
58	M	21	78	92	9.0	76	85	-		1.4	4	0	6	
59	M	19	80	97	10.4	90	95	-	3225	1.6	-	3	4	
60	M	30			10.8	80		-	2640	1.9	+	1	5	
61	M	14	71	92	9.7	93	109	-	1995	<1.2	+	2	20	Corneal erosion
62	M	17	79	98	10.9	99	101	-	3225	3.4	+	2	2	
63	F	29	88	96	11.2	84	89	-	3730	1.2	16	2	8	
64	F	33	87	93	12.8	91	103	-	3535	1.5	13	4	7	
65	M	8	70	101	7.9	93	89	-			0	R	6	
66	Post-measles		died											
67	M	23							2910	4.1	1	R	10	
68	F	30			10.9	80					3	2	8	died.
69	F	27	78	87	9.5	74	90	-	3330	2.5	3	1	8	
70	F	42	94	96	12.7	85	91	-	2830	1.6	8	3	7	
71	F	20	70	84	7.2	62	81	+	1900	1.4	0	6	5	
72	F	72	111	96	18.3	86	97	-	3370	1.5	3	1	6	
73	F	13							2455	1.2	13	3	5	died
74	F	13	70	92	10.0	98	112	+			1	6	7	
75	F	42	95	95	12.3	79	87		2545	1.2	19	3	6	
76		9									+	2	4	
77	F	17	74	92	9.5	86	99		3790	2.4	-	4	3	
78		8	64	92	7.2	86	104				+	4	4	
79		18	75	92	9.4	83	92	-	4120	2.5	+	3	7	
80	F	18	72	88				-	1900	1.4	0	2	10	

Nr	Sex	Age	H	H/A	W	W/A	W/H	Vacc	Alb	RBP	Ker	Adm	Obser	Remarks
81	F	156	151	96	45.5	101	115	-	3040	1.8	-	1	2	
82		11	64	87	7.0	73	101	-			20	4	8	
83	F	8	59	85	6.1	73	114	+	2410	1.7	1	1	8	
84	F	24	80	92	9.9	80	90	+	4200	2.7	8	R	8	
85	F	30	83	9o	10.2	76	89	+			0	2	6	
86	M	13	78	103	9.5	93	90	+			1	2	8	
87	M	8	57	82	4.3	52	100	-	3225	<1.2	2	2	7	
88	F	13	70	91	8.8	85	99	-	3265	1.4	17	1	6	
89	F	7	61	90	7.0	87	123	-	4320	1.8	1	2	5	
90	M	18	74	91	8.7	77	91	-	2220	1.2	8	3	14	
91	M	24	80	92	9.7	78	88	+			0	3	5	
92	M	8	65	94	7.4	88	107	-	3040	2.0	5	3	15	
93	M	14	71	92	9.2	88	103	-	3775	1.5	2	1	7	
94	M	29	95	104	11.2	84	79	-			11	1	13	
95	F	49	95	92	13.2	80	93	-	3580	2.7	0	1	6	
96	M	108						-	3375	2.3	7	2	8	
97	F	1o8			22.5	78		-	2725	1.7	7	1	9	
98	Post-measles													
99	M	28	80	88	11.1	85	101		2635	1.4	5	1	13	
100	F	28	85	94	12.2	93	117	-	3375	1.3	5	2	9	
101	M	27	80	89	11.2	87	102	-	3570	3.3	2	1	8	
102	F	24							2545	<1.2	+	2	1	died
103	F	25	72	82	11.1	88	119				0	2	9	
104	F	38									1	1	6	
105	F	9	65	92	8.1	91	117	-	3525	<1.2	0	4	10	
106	F	12	76	102	9.3	94	91	-	2175	2.1	4	R	14	
107	F	10	62	86	6.2	67	98	-			-	R	4	died
108	F	24	82	94	8.3	67	73	-	2590	1.5	5	1	7	
109	F	38	88	90	10.6	72	84	-		1.8	14	1	8	
110	M	28	79	87	9.4	72	87	-	1840	1.2	17	1	8	
111	M	120	144	104	32.5	100	92		3040	2.7	0	1	5	
112	Non·existent.													
113	F	36	87	91	11.3	78	91	-	2715	1.2	2	1	9	Corneal erosion
114	M	66	102	89	18.4	89	114		2800	1.6	1	1	9	
115	M	36	85	89	12.1	83	101	-	2305	<1.2	0	1	6	
116	F	22	Malnutrition						3375	1.5	0	1	19	
117	M	66	104	91	16.2	78	98	-	2790	1.6	1	1	10	Exposure Ulcer
118	F	42	92	92	11.2	72	83	-	2500	1.2	2	1	9	
119	F	31							3040	2.4	6	2	9	
120	F	13	66	87	7.8	76	105	-	2995	<1.2	10	3	16	

Nr	Sex	Age	H	H/A	W	W/A	W/H	Vacc	Alb	RBP	Ker	Adm	Obser	Remarks
121	M	14	73	95	9.0	87	94	-	2625	<1.2	6	2	10	
122	No measles													
123	F	27	82	91	10.4	81	91	-	3175	1.2	1	1	10	
124	M	5	57	89	5.9	86	123	-	3040	1.7	15	1	8	
125	M	96	126	97	27.4	99	106	-	3720	1.6	0	R	6	
126	F	76	118	99	19.8	88	88		1795	1.2	0	3	9	
127	M	168							2995	2.4	6	1	7	
128	M	25	82	93	11.9	94	104	+			2	1	9	
129	F	81	108	91	15.8	68	88	-	2785		15	R	17	
130	F	18	80	98	8.6	76	79	-	2820	1.2	19	R	11	
131	M	15	78	100	11.3	107	107	-			2	1	7	
132	F	68	106	94	14.9	75	87	+	4120	1.4	8	1	7	
133	F	7	60	89	7.1	89	125				1	3	9	
134	M	17	81	101	10.0	91	88	-	3480	2.4	12	R	9	
135	M	21	80	95	9.9	83	91	-			6	-3	15	
136	F	23	85	98	10.3	84	86	-	3150	2.9	1	1	7	
137	M	32						-	3480	3.0	1	R	6	
138	F	18	80	98	9.1	81	83	-	3150	1.7	1	1	15	
139	F	17	68	84	8.6	78	108	-			2	1	9	
140	F	84	117	96	25.0	105	115	-	3300	2.5	0	6	13	
141	M	60	103	93	15.0	77	91	-	3295	2.6	8	1	9	
142	F	9	66	93	6.7	75	91	-	3740	1.2	0	6	13	
143	F	15	65	83	6.1	58	85	-			+		2	died
144	F	44	94	93	12.2	77	87	+			3	1	8	
145	F	31	82	89	8.1	59	71	-			1	4	11	
146	M	10	66	91	6.4	69	86	-			6	1	6	
147	F	60	99	91	17.6	96	115	-	3580	2.8	12	4	9	
148	F	21	79	94	9.0	76	83	-	2770	<1.2	3	1	9	
149	M	18	75	92	9.0	80	90	-	3390	2.4	11	3	9	died, corneal erosion
150	F	15	63	81	8.1	76	125	-			9	-1	8	
151	M	23	81	94	10.4	85	94	-			-	R	7	
152	M	8	64	92	6.5	77	96	-	2910	1.2	4	3	5	
153	Post Measles													
154	F	44	96	95	15.0	95	103	-		1.7	13	4	5	
155	M	91	Malnutrition						1960	<1.2	+	2	1	died

Curriculum vitae

N.W.H.M. Dekkers

31-12-1940   geboren te Tilburg

05-07-1958   Eindexamen Gymnasium β aan het St. Odulphuslyceum te Tilburg

06-04-1964   Doctoraal examen Geneeskunde aan de Katholieke Universiteit Nijmegen. Hierna volgde Co-assistentschappen aan de Stichting Klinisch Hoger Onderwijs te Rotterdam. Na een vakantie-assistentschap psychiatrie (Prof. Dr. J.A. Ladee) werd de opleiding tot arts 22-03-1967 afgesloten met het artsexamen te Leiden. De militaire dienst werd doorgebracht bij de Koninklijke Luchtmacht in W. Duitsland, 's-Gravenhage en Gilze-Rijen, waarna een paar jaar waarrťeming in de huisartsen-praktijk volgde.

01-06-1972   Aanvang opleiding tot oogarts aan het Oogziekenhuis te Rotterdam, onder Prof. Dr. H.E. Henkes en Prof. Dr. A.Th.M. van Balen. Deze opleiding werd van 01-11-1974 tot 15-07-1978 onderbroken voor het gaan leiden van een groot oogheelkundig project van de Prof. Weve Stichting in W. Kenya, waar ook de basis van dit proefschrift werd gelegd.

15-07-1979   Volgde de inschrijving in het Specialisten Register als oogarts.

01-10-1979   Vestiging als oogarts in Tilburg aan het St. Elisabeth Ziekenhuis.